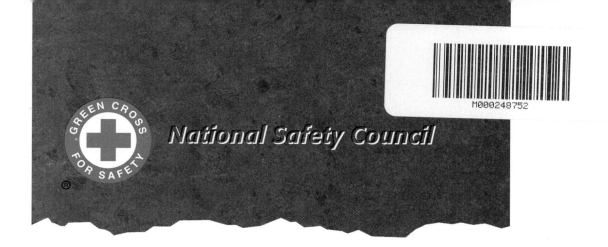

National Safety Council

FIRST AID AND CPR FOR INFANTS AND CHILDREN

THIRD EDITION

JONES AND BARTLETT PUBLISHERS

Sudbury, Massachusetts

BOSTON   TORONTO   LONDON   SINGAPORE

World Headquarters
Jones and Bartlett Publishers
40 Tall Pine Drive, Sudbury, MA 01776
978-443-5000
nsc@jbpub.com, Internet: http://www.jbpub.com/nsc

Jones and Bartlett Publishers Canada
P.O. Box 19020, Toronto, ON M5S 1X1, CANADA

Jones and Bartlett Publishers International
Barb House, Barb Mews
London W6 7PA, UK

The CPR procedures in this book are based on the most current recommendations of responsible medical sources. The National Safety Council and the publisher, however, make no guarantee as to, and assume no responsibility for the correctness, sufficiency or completeness of such information or recommendations. Other or additional safety measures may be required under particular circumstances.

Library of Congress Cataloging-in-Publication Data
First aid and CPR : infants and children / National Safety Council. —3rd ed.
    p.   cm.
  Includes index.
  ISBN 0-7637-0633-7
    1. Pediatric emergencies.   2. First aid in illness and injury.
  3. CPR (First aid) for children.   4. CPR (First aid) for infants.
  I. National Safety Council.
  RJ370.F57   1998
  618.92'0025—dc21   97-41585
                                                             CIP

Emergency Care Editor: Tracy Murphy Foss
Emergency Care Associate Editor: Nancy Carosella
Senior Production Editor: Cynthia Knowles Maciel

Illustrations: Rolin Graphics
Typesetting and Prepress: Clarinda Company
Cover Photographs: Center, ©Index Stock Photography and/or Richard Wood 1998; clockwise from top left, ©Ken Fisher/Tony Stone Images, ©Zephyr Images, ©Index Stock Photography and/or Dave Lissy 1998, ©Mark Gibson
Printing and Binding: Banta Company

Printed in the United States of America
02 01 00 99   10 9 8 7 6 5 4 3 2

Contents

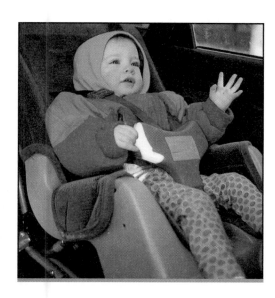

Contents

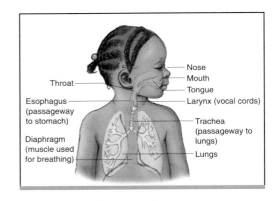

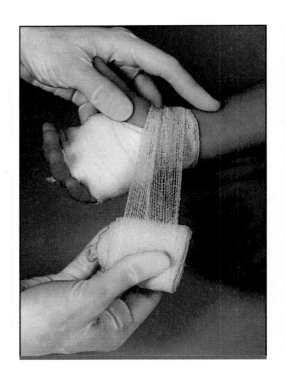

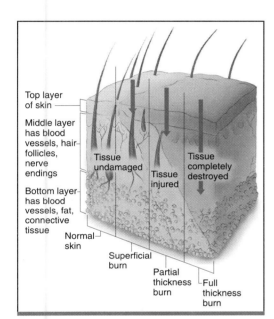

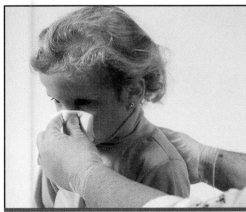

Caring for a nosebleed

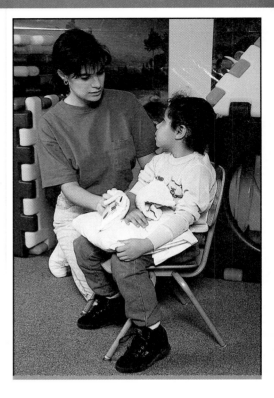

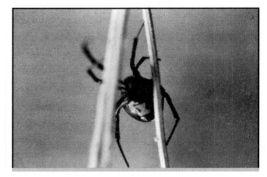

Black widow spider

Contents

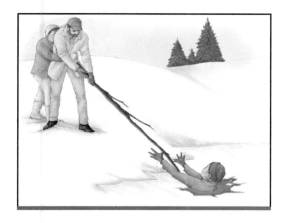

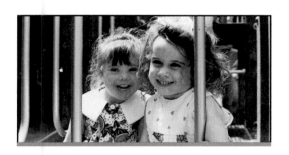

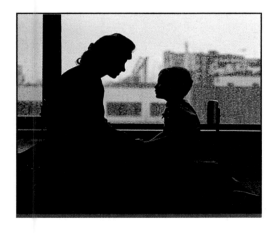

Contents

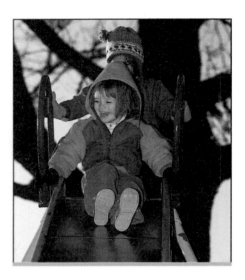

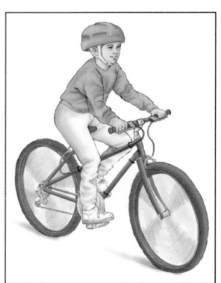

About the National Safety Council Program

Congratulations on selecting the National Safety Council's First Aid and CPR program! You join good company, as the National Safety Council has successfully trained over 2 million people worldwide in first aid and cardiopulmonary resuscitation (CPR). The National Safety Council's training network of nearly 10,000 instructors at over 2,500 sites worldwide has established the National Safety Council programs as the standard by which all others are judged.

In setting the standards, the National Safety Council has worked in close cooperation with hundreds of national and international organizations, thousands of corporations, thousands of leading educators, dozens of leading medical organizations, and hundreds of state and local governmental agencies. Their collective input has helped create programs that stand alone in quality. Consider just a few of the National Safety Council's current collaborations:

World's Leading Medical Organizations

The National Safety Council is currently working with both the American Academy of Orthopaedic Surgeons (AAOS) and the Wilderness Medical Society (WMS) to help bring innovative, new training programs to the marketplace. The National Safety Council and the AAOS are developing a new First Responder program and the National Safety Council and the WMS are developing the first-of-its-kind wilderness first aid program.

United States Government

The National Safety Council has developed an innovative computer-based training program for first aid that is currently being used to train United States Postal Service employees.

World's Leading Corporations

Thousands of corporations including Westinghouse, Disney, Exxon, General Motors, Pacific Bell, Ameritech, and U.S. West have selected many of the National Safety Council emergency care programs to train employees.

World's Leading Colleges and Universities

Hundreds of leading colleges and universities are working closely with the National Safety Council to fully develop and implement the Internet Initiative that will establish the National Safety Council as the leading on-line provider of emergency care programs.

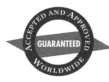

Most importantly, in selecting the National Safety Council programs, you can feel confident that the programs are accepted and approved worldwide. You can rely on the National Safety Council. Founded in 1913, the National Safety Council is dedicated to protecting life, promoting health, and reducing accidental death. For more than 80 years, the National Safety Council has been the world's leading authority on safety/injury education.

 National Safety Council

Acknowledgments

Principal Authors

Stephanie L. O'Neill, B.S., R.N.
O'Neill-Page, Inc.
Belmont, MA

Constance Q. Page, B.A., R.N.
O'Neill-Page, Inc.
Belmont, MA

Reviewers

The National Safety Council would like to thank the following individuals for their efforts in reviewing the complete manuscript or selected chapters of this text and its previous edition.

Deborah Z. Altschuler
National Pediculosis Association
Newton, MA

Betty Jane Evans
Dade County Citizens Safety Council
Miami, FL

Margaret Anderson
Pfizer Central Research Division
Gorton, CT

Linda Gosselin
MECTA
Milbury, MA

Carol Bufton
Minnesota National Safety Council
St. Paul, MN

Mary Horne
Children's Hospital
Boston, MA

Ann Coley
Sumter Area Technical College
Sumter, SC

Barbara Jacobs
Boston Head Start, ABCD, Inc.
Boston, MA

Richard Cooper
SEMTA
Rye, NH

Claudella Jones
The National Institute for Burn Medicine
Ann Arbor, MI

Susan Denton
Central Florida Safety Council
Orlando, FL

Sandra Lewis
Sandra Lewis Training Associates
So. Easton, MA

Barbara Miller
First Responder
Laguna Nigel, CA

Paula Mitchell
Child Health Alert
Newton Highlands, MA

Cindy Pasquarello
Joslin Diabetic Center
Boston, MA

Jodi Rupe
Texas Safety Council
Austin, TX

R. Lorraine Samuel
Cambridge School Department
Cambridge, MA

Barbara Seabolt
Comprehensive Health and Safety
Education
Farmington, MI

Bob Sklar
MST FastPro
Orange, CA

Linda Softley
Massachusetts Poison Control Center
Boston, MA

Rose Ann Soloway
National Capital Poison Center
Washington, D.C.

Gina Stanke
Children's Mercy Hospital
Kansas City, MO

Alton Thygerson
Brigham Young University
Provo, UT

Judy Walker
Harvard University Child Care
Cambridge, MA

John Ward
North Alabama Chapter Safety Council
Birmingham, AL

Kathleen Zents
Safety & Health Council of Western
Missouri & Kansas
Kansas City, MO

We would like to thank the following programs for their cooperation with the photographs:

Action for Boston Community Development, Inc./South End Head Start Program
Charlestown, Massachusetts Head Start/Day Care Program

We would also like to thank the children and teachers who so generously posed for us.

CHAPTER 1

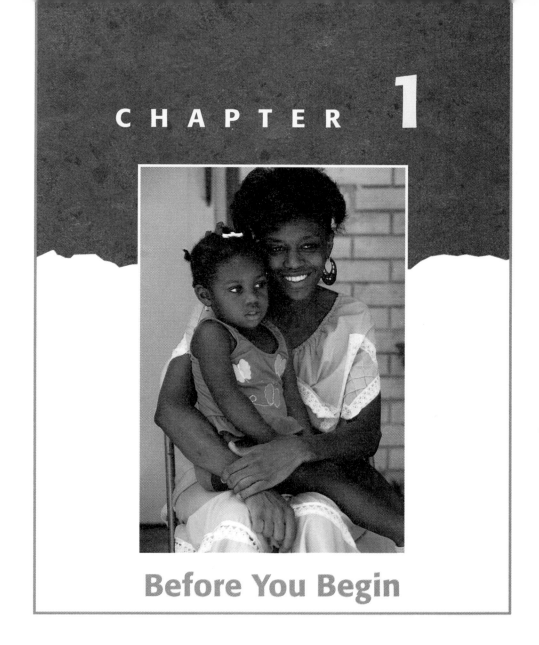

Before You Begin

We all know how wonderful it is to be greeted by a young child's smile and a hug or to be shown a special piece of artwork by its proud creator, and there are few experiences warmer than holding a child on your lap while you read a favorite story. Despite the runny noses, diapers, spilled milk, and the other less attractive tasks that are part of your day, the emotional rewards of child care are tremendously satisfying.

As a child care provider, you have the important job of caring for and nurturing young children. You make sure that children are served well-balanced meals, have art materials for creating wonderful projects, spend part of every day in outdoor play, and get the rest they need. You expose them to literature, and you answer their many questions about why things are the way they are. From you, they learn why it is important to share and to be kind.

In addition to the nurturing aspects of your work, you must be thinking constantly about the safety of children. Ordinary adult habits—such as leaving a purse on the floor, setting a pair of scissors on the counter, placing a cup of hot coffee on the kitchen table, keeping vitamins at the bathroom sink, or leaving a second-story window open—present potentially dangerous situations for children. The protective environment you create and your influence and example help to guide children safely in their development toward becoming creative, self-assured, and considerate people.

Injuries: The #1 Health Problem for Children

In the United States, unintentional injuries are the leading health problem for children between ages 1 and 16. According to the National Safety Council, injuries cause more deaths among children than all diseases combined and are the leading cause of disability. Each year, an estimated 600,000 children are hospitalized for injuries and almost 16 million are seen in emergency medical facilities for treatment.

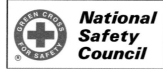

National Safety Council

The Centers for Disease Control estimates that more than 30,000 children suffer permanent disabilities from injuries each year. These disabilities have enormous adverse effects on a child's development and future productivity and severely strain the financial and emotional resources of families.

The Need for Injury Prevention Education

Unintentional injuries are often referred to as accidents, because they occur unexpectedly and seem uncontrollable. In fact, however, many occurrences referred to as accidents are better termed "preventable" injuries. They can be avoided if a few simple injury-prevention steps are practiced consistently. Unfortunately, injuries occur if these steps are ignored.

Consider the injury that results when a young child swallows a cleaning product that was not properly stored or when a toddler falls down a flight of stairs that did not have a stairway gate in place. Such preventable injuries threaten the health and safety of children who cannot yet protect themselves and leave the responsible adult with regrets, worry, and guilt.

Public education and awareness programs have had a positive effect on the reduction of childhood injuries and deaths. Thousands more could be avoided every year through currently available prevention strategies. For example:

- The enactment of state seat belt laws and child safety restraint laws, plus the efforts to reduce drunk driving, have contributed to the reduction of vehicle-related injuries and deaths.

- Public awareness concerning the use of smoke detectors has reduced injuries and deaths that result from home fires.

- Product safety testing on juvenile products has significantly reduced injuries to young children.

- The proper use of bicycle helmets has reduced the number and severity of head injuries.

- Educational programs for preschool and elementary school children concerning fire prevention, poison prevention, motor vehicle restraints, and water safety have all contributed to a decrease in the number of injuries to children.

However, even our best injury-prevention strategies cannot prevent all mishaps. When a child's bicycle tire hits a rock and the child falls, skinning an elbow or breaking an arm, it is still, and always will be, an unpreventable accident that is part of the passage through childhood.

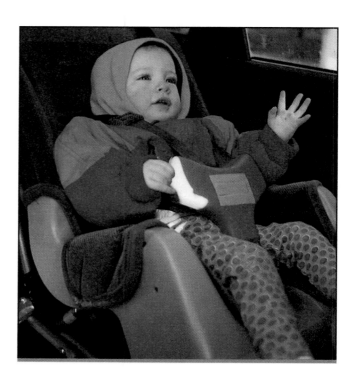

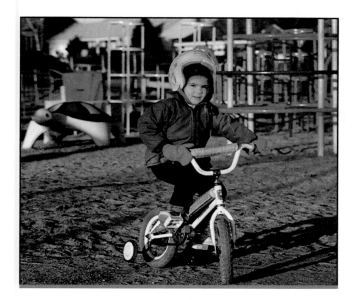

An awareness of which dangers can, and frequently do, cause injuries and knowledge about how you can make your child's environment safer are important components of injury prevention for children. Injury prevention steps can reduce the likelihood that you will need to use your first aid skills.

What Is First Aid?

First aid is the immediate care given to an injured or suddenly ill person. It provides temporary assistance until medical care, if needed, is obtained. In fact, most injuries and sudden illnesses require no more than first aid care. However, proper first aid can also mean the difference between life and death, rapid and slow recovery, or temporary and permanent disability.

The Need for First Aid Training

Injuries can occur no matter how caring and watchful adults are and despite the best of safety plans. Because of the frequency of injury to children, it is likely that a child care provider will, at some time, be present when an injury or sudden illness occurs. The types of injuries that happen to children often directly relate to the child's age and developmental level. (Refer to *Common Injuries Related to Child's Developmental Level* in Chapter 17). Planning to prevent these injuries is essential, and it is equally essential to master first aid techniques.

Legal Aspects of First Aid

No one is required to provide first aid unless a legal obligation to do so exists. For example, even a physician can ignore a stranger who is experiencing a seizure or who has a broken leg. Moral obligations exist but they are not the same as legal obligations.

A person has a legal responsibility to act in the following situations:

- **When employment requires it.** The responsibility for the safety of other people is inherent in some jobs, such as police officer, lifeguard, chauffeur, teacher, and child care provider.
- **In a pre-existing relationship.** When there is a pre-existing relationship between two people, such as parent and child or an adult driver with a child in the vehicle, it is understood that the adult in these situations has a responsibility to provide or to obtain first aid care, if necessary.

In addition, once a person begins treating a child for an injury, the care giver must not stop until relieved by another competent adult who can seek further appropriate treatment, or until emergency medical help arrives, or until the care giver is physically exhausted.

First Aid Program Standards

Delivering high quality first aid care is necessary, and maintaining standards in the training of first aiders is essential. The National Safety Council first aid and cardiopulmonary resuscitation (CPR) programs meet the requirements of state regulations and follow current first aid procedures and practices as established by national emergency care and safety-related organizations. A trained first aider should provide appropriate care only within the scope of this training.

Obtaining Permission to Give First Aid

A person should always obtain permission before giving first aid. Most child care centers require parents to complete forms that provide a medical history and permission to have the child treated in an emergency situation.

In the event that the injured child is unknown to you, permission must first be obtained from the parent or guardian. Verbal consent is acceptable. Tell the parent that you are trained in first aid and explain what you plan to do. If a parent or guardian is not available, emergency lifesaving first aid may be given without consent, because it is assumed that the child's parent would consent in this instance.

Combative older children who threaten to harm themselves or others can present a difficult management problem. Remember that, although infrequently needed, police officers have the authority to restrain and transport a child as well as an adult.

When a Parent Refuses to Give Permission for First Aid

Rarely, a first aider encounters a parent who refuses to give permission to give first aid to a seriously injured or ill child. When this does occur, it is usually done on the basis of moral, ethical, or religious grounds. If a parent refuses to give permission, make every effort to convince him or her of the need for first aid. If the parent remains unconvinced, call for emergency medical help and allow professionals to deal with the situation.

The Good Samaritan Laws

Although they vary from state to state, almost every state has Good Samaritan laws designed to protect medical personnel who, in an emergency situation, give aid to a person who is injured or becomes ill suddenly. Some states have broadened these laws to include trained first aiders, to encourage them to step forward in an emergency. The first aider should act in good faith and in a responsible manner, follow accepted first aid guidelines, act without compensation, and perform without gross negligence or malicious misconduct.

Infection Prevention When Giving First Aid

Most people are aware of the concern over serious and life-threatening illnesses that can be passed from one person to another. They feel hesitant to risk their own health for the sake of a stranger. It is only normal to have these worries.

Knowing how germs are transmitted from person to person and how to protect yourself from disease while giving first aid care will enable you to act wisely and with confidence.

Take Steps Now . . .

1. Post emergency telephone numbers, including the poison control center, next to every telephone.
2. Keep a well-stocked first aid kit in your home or child care center and another one for travel. Routinely check and replace products that have been used or have expired.
3. Be sure all staff members know first aid and CPR. Check your state's requirements by contacting your state's licensing agency.
4. Have disposable gloves available in several easy-to-reach locations.
5. Be sure your child care center's name or your house number is clearly posted outside.
6. Check the batteries in smoke detectors in the spring and fall when you change your clocks.
7. Make sure your child care center has a fire escape plan, including a meeting spot outside. Practice this plan with the children and all staff members.
8. Make sure all adults know the location of fire extinguishers. Do not store them near a stove, oven, or other location where you might need to use it, because you might not be able to reach it when there is a fire.
9. Always have passengers in your car buckle their seat belts. Ask parents to transport their children to your center or home in an age-appropriate child safety restraint.

We are all exposed to germs every day in our homes, work places, and schools—wherever people are together. And when people are together, the spread of illness is to be expected. The best known illness-causing germs, or microorganisms, are bacteria and viruses. Although not all bacteria and viruses cause illness, a small number do and some of them can be deadly.

Infections caused by bacteria, such as strep throat and many ear infections, are treated with antibiotics. Infections caused by viruses, such as the common cold and chicken pox, have no specific medicines to cure them. There are medicines available to relieve the unpleasant symptoms of a viral infection, but the body must rely on its immune system to destroy a virus. Unfortunately, a few viruses cannot be subdued by the immune system and can destroy it, threatening the life of the individual. The human immunodeficiency virus (HIV), which causes AIDS, and the hepatitis B and C viruses behave in this way.

Organisms that cause disease enter the body in one of four ways: touching, ingesting, inhaling, and through blood-to-blood exchange. When giving first aid care, you can reduce your risk of contracting or transmitting disease by following these guidelines:

- Wear disposable gloves when providing first aid care.

- If disposable gloves are not available, use another barrier, such as a thickly-folded towel, a plastic bag, or several thick layers of gauze pads. Plastic wrap placed over the gauze or towel increases the effective- ness of the barrier.

- Wash your hands immedi- ately after removing dispos- able gloves. Use antimicrobial wipes if hand-washing facili- ties are unavailable.

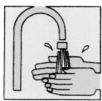

DO NOT

- **touch blood or other body fluids with un- gloved hands.**
- **touch clothing or other articles soiled by blood or body fluids with ungloved hands.**
- **blow on a wound in an attempt to soothe pain.**
- **eat or drink while giving first aid.**
- **touch your eyes, nose, or mouth with your hands while giving first aid.**

Be Prepared with First Aid Supplies

Although you may hope an emergency never occurs, you need to be prepared for one. Part of being prepared means keeping a well-stocked first aid kit. With all necessary supplies on hand, you are better able to act quickly and efficiently when an emergency arises.

Store all supplies in a locked container out of the reach of children. Plastic tool or tackle boxes make good containers for first aid supplies because they are lightweight, sturdy, portable, and close se- curely. Keep the container in a cool, dry location. Make sure all staff (or family) members (and chil- dren, if they are old enough to retrieve it) know

where the kit is stored. Remember to take your traveling first aid kit along on a field trip. It is also a good idea to keep a first aid kit in your car for your personal or family use.

Antibiotics and other medicines prescribed for a child's illness should not be stored in a first aid kit. Many of these medicines must be refrigerated. Check the first aid kit regularly for items that have been used and not replaced. Discard expired items.

The supplies that you should have in your first aid kit include the following:

Adhesive bandages (assorted sizes)

Antimicrobial hand wipes (for use when hand- washing facilities are unavailable)

Alcohol wipes

Blanket

CPR mouth-to-barrier device (child and infant sizes)

Commercial cold pack

Cotton swabs

Disposable gloves

Eye pads

Gauze pads (assorted sizes)

Measuring spoons

Nonstick sterile pads (assorted sizes)

Paper cups

Pencil and paper

Petroleum jelly

Rolled elastic bandages (assorted sizes)

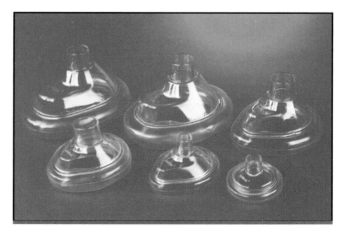

Disposable mouth-to-barrier devices like these come in several sizes. Shown here, from front right clockwise, are sizes for the neonate, infant, toddler, large adult, medium adult, and small adult/child.

Rolled gauze bandages (assorted sizes)

Safety pins

Sam™ splints

Soap (antibacterial liquid)

Syrup of ipecac

Scissors

Sling or triangular bandages

Tape (adhesive or other first aid types)

Thermometer (digital)

Tongue depressor

Tweezers

White cotton handkerchief (for removing floating objects from eye)

Triangular bandages

In addition, you might want to include the items below. Know your center's policies regarding the use of these products.

Acetaminophen

Baking soda

Calamine lotion

Oil of cloves (for a toothache)

Topical antibiotic ointments

An emergency self-treatment kit for allergies, if prescribed by a physician for a specific child in your center, should be kept in your first aid kit.

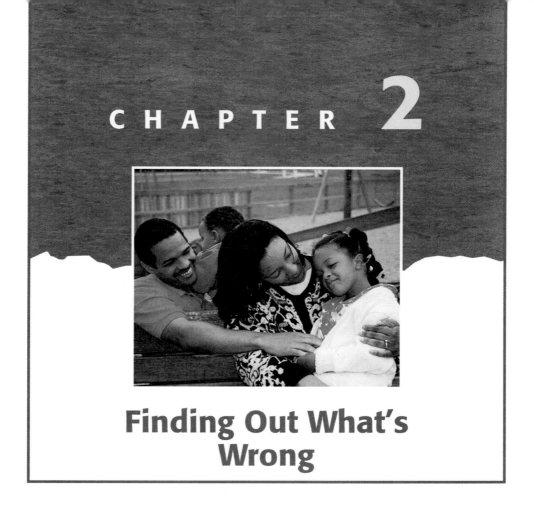

CHAPTER 2

Finding Out What's Wrong

During an emergency in which a child is involved, it is essential to remain calm and in control. A calm attitude and methodical approach inspires the confidence of an injured child and sets a standard for other adults to follow.

First aiders should avoid making an injury worse by their own actions. To that end, always handle an injured child gently and avoid any unnecessary movements that might aggravate an undetected fracture or spine injury.

Scene Survey

When an injury occurs, take a moment and let your eyes help you figure out what might have happened and how to proceed.

- **Scan the injury scene to make sure that it is safe for you to approach.** In most situations in which a child is injured, there will be no hazards to your safety. However, if there are, do not risk making yourself another victim. For instance, be alert for unusual dangers, such as deep water, downed electrical wires, or chemical fumes. Before you can begin to help an injured person, you might need to call the electric company to turn off the current or the fire department to evaluate toxic fumes.
- **Look around to gather clues** about what might have happened. For instance, there might be a child lying on the ground beside an overturned ladder or underneath an open second-story window.
- **Check the scene for more than one injured child.**

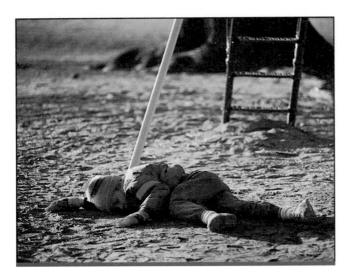

Look around to gather clues.

Primary Survey: Checking for Life-Threatening Injuries

Perform the primary survey to find life-threatening problems that must be attended to immediately. Most injuries do not involve life-threatening situations. Therefore, in most instances, it will take only moments to complete the primary survey. To begin:

- **Check responsiveness.** If the child does not respond when called by name or gently tapped on the shoulder, assume that the child is unconscious. If the injured child does respond, see *Checking for Other Injuries.*

- **Send someone to call for emergency medical help** if the child is unresponsive or appears to have a serious injury.

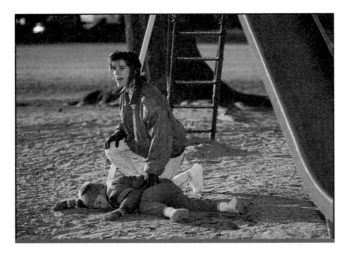

Shout for help and send someone to call for emergency medical help.

- **Position unresponsive child on back.** Avoid any twisting motion by rolling the head, neck, and spine as a unit. Check for the most vital information using the letters "ABCD" to help you remember the following steps:

- **Airway:** Is the airway open? The passageway connecting the nose and mouth to the lungs must be open for air to pass through. If an unconscious child is positioned flat on the back, the airway can become blocked by the tongue. Tilting the head backward slightly moves the tongue out of the airway. Sometimes a foreign object is the cause of a blocked airway.

- **Breathing:** Is the child breathing? Breathing supplies oxygen to the heart muscle. When breathing stops, the heart continues to beat for only a few minutes before it, too, stops. To determine if the child is breathing, use the look, listen, and feel skills discussed in Chapter 3.

- **Circulation:** Is a pulse present? If the pulse is not present, the heart is not beating. If the heart is not beating, no other body function, including breathing can work. A second concern relating to circulation is severe bleeding. Is severe bleeding present? Is clothing blood-soaked or is blood spurting from a deep wound? Severe bleeding interferes with the effectiveness of CPR.

If there is a problem with any one of the "ABCs," stop and treat these life-threatening problems before going on with your assessment.

- Disability
  Damage to the spine: If damage to the spine is suspected, such as after a fall from a ladder that has caused unconsciousness or after a motor vehicle accident, tell the child not to move, or move the child only as much as is necessary to check the ABCs and perform the care necessary, because any change of position might make the spine injury worse.

Checking for Other Injuries

Check for other injuries only after you are certain that the child is conscious and breathing. This is when you locate and prioritize additional injuries that do not pose an immediate threat to life but that might become life-threatening if left untreated. Often an injury is obvious, such as bleeding or swelling, but you must not assume that the obvious injuries are the only injuries. Most injuries are accompanied by pain and abnormal function.

Deformity
open wounds
Tenderness
Swelling

look for in
fractures, then

Circulation
Sensation
movement

Find Out

Help the child to calm down by speaking to the child in a comforting manner. Use short sentences and familiar words. Ask other adults and children if they saw what happened. Reassure the child by explaining that you will help. If you are caring for a child that you do not know, obtain the parent's permission, if possible, before beginning first aid. See Chapter 1 for information on obtaining permission.

Ask simple, nonthreatening questions such as, "Tell me what happened," and, "Point to where it hurts." Try to be as honest as possible. You might not know the extent of the injuries, but you can say, "You are safe now," and "I am taking good care of you." The word SAMPLE can help you remember other important information that might be needed at a later time by emergency medical personnel.

S: Signs and symptoms are what you observe and the child's complaints.

A: Allergies might give a clue as to the problem.

M: Medications might give a clue as to the problem.

P: Pre-existing illness means a known health condition relating to the problem.

L: Last food or beverage should be known, in case surgery is needed or food poisoning is suspected.

E: Events before the injury, such as a child on playground equipment or eating.

Always check for a medical alert tag on a child who is unknown to you. The tag is worn as a necklace or a bracelet. It provides important information about allergies, medications, and pre-existing illness and a 24-hour emergency telephone number. Never remove a child's medical alert tag.

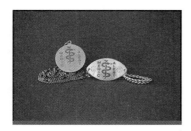
Medical alert tag

Physical Examination: A Head-to-Toe Check

Checking the child from head to toe is necessary only if the child's injury is the result of a forceful impact. An example of a situation in which a child

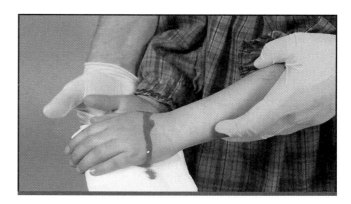
A sign

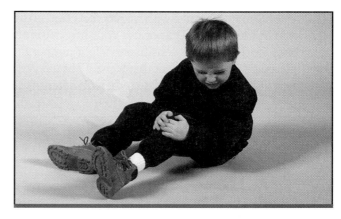
A symptom

might be seriously injured are a fall from a tree limb or a bicycle accident. Minor injuries do not require a complete head-to-toe check.

As you examine the child, look for important signs and symptoms of injury. A *sign* is a condition that the first aider sees, hears, or feels, such as a pale face, difficulty breathing, or cool skin. A *symptom* is a condition that the child feels and describes to the first aider, such as nausea or back pain.

Explain what you are doing and why. Removing clothing is usually not necessary. Always handle an injured child gently and as little as possible. Avoid any unnecessary movements that might aggravate an undetected fracture or spine injury. Examine the part that hurts last.

Skin Color

A blue or gray color around a child's lips and nose in a light-skinned child is easily noticed and indicates that the child is having a problem breathing. In a dark-skinned child, however, color changes are not as easily seen. For any skin type, color changes can best be seen by looking at the nailbeds or the mucous membrane inside the mouth and the lower eyelids. Healthy mucous membranes are moist and pink because of their many blood vessels. Mucous membranes that do not have enough oxygen appear pale to blue or gray.

Breathing

Once the child has calmed down, notice if breathing seems difficult. Is the child breathing comfortably or does breathing cause pain or discomfort? Does the child use abdominal muscles to breathe or do the nostrils flare?

Temperature

You can get some idea of the child's temperature by touching the back of your hand to the child's cheek, chest, or abdomen. A child with a fever feels unusually warm in these areas. Do not use your fingertips or palm because they are not sensitive to slight temperature differences. If you suspect that a child has a fever, take the child's temperature using a thermometer.

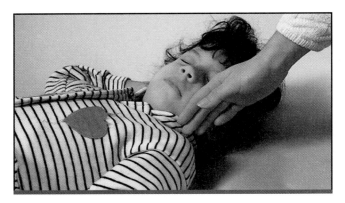

Checking body temperature

Head

Check the scalp for a bleeding wound, swelling, or depressions. Does the child complain of pain?

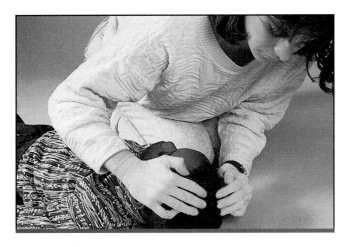

Checking the head

Taking care not to move the head, check the ears and nose for clear fluid or bloody drainage. Look in the mouth for blood or foreign objects, such as gum, candy, food, or small toy pieces.

Eyes

Gently separate the eyelids and look at the pupils, the small dark center of the eye. Normally, pupils become smaller when exposed to light. If pupils are unequal in size, the child might have experienced an internal head injury. Large or dilated pupils might indicate shock or internal bleeding. Pupils that are constricted might indicate a drug overdose or poisoning.

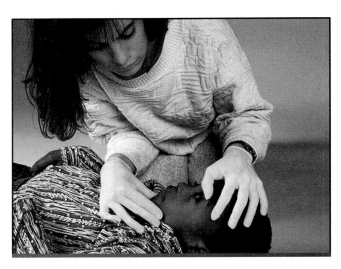

Checking the pupils

Spine

Tell the child not to move. If you suspect the child has suffered a spine injury, ask if the child feels any pain or tingling in the arms or legs. Check the sensation, or feeling, and strength in the arms and legs by asking the child to press each foot against your hand and to squeeze your fingers with each hand.

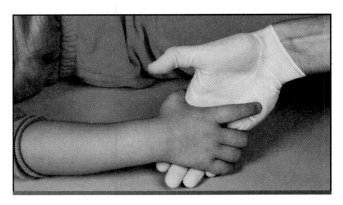

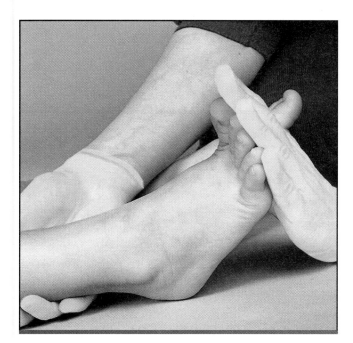

Checking for a spine injury

Chest

Check for cuts, bruises, penetrations, pain, or unusual positioning of the shoulders and ribs.

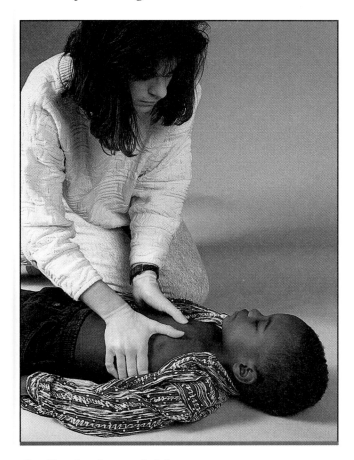

Checking the chest and abdomen

Abdomen

Gently feel the abdomen to check for pain and involuntary tightening of the stomach muscles, called "guarding."

Arms and Legs

Check the arms and legs for bleeding, deformity, and pain. Compare one side of the body to the other. The child should be able to move and feel the fingers and toes. The hands and feet should be warm to the touch.

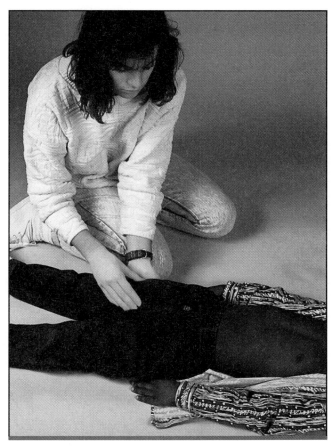

Checking the legs

Emergency Moves When Damage to the Spine Is Suspected

These emergency moves are to be used when moving an unresponsive child or a child whom you suspect might have damage to the spine away from a life-threatening location. For example, a child must be moved when lying near flames, near a car that might explode, near a wall that might collapse, or in an environment of toxic fumes.

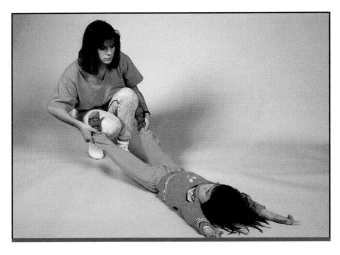

Ankle drag. Firmly grasp the child's ankles and pull the child away from danger. Use this method only on smooth surfaces.

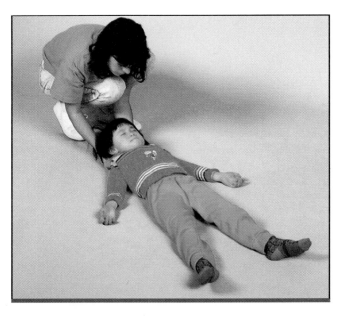

Clothing drag. Firmly grasp clothing around the collar and support the child's head on your wrists while pulling the child away from danger. Use this method to support the child's neck over rough terrain.

Positioning an Injured Child

When a serious injury occurs, proper positioning makes a child more comfortable, reduces the risk of further injury, and helps prevent the child's condition from worsening. Position the child according to the injuries you find and the child's complaints.

Recovery Position

Use this position for a child who is unresponsive yet breathing and for any child who is vomiting.

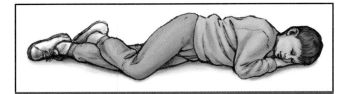

Recovery position

Roll the child onto the left side as one unit. Place the back of the child's right hand under the left cheek. Bend the right knee slightly and place the right leg over and in front of the left leg. This position stabilizes and prevents the child from rolling forward or backward. It keeps the airway open and reduces the risk of the child choking on vomit.

Raised Head and Shoulders Position

Use this position if the child is experiencing difficulty breathing or has a head injury, but do not use this position if you suspect a neck or spine injury. Elevate the head and shoulders so that the child is in a semi-sitting position, which makes breathing easier and creates less pressure inside the skull.

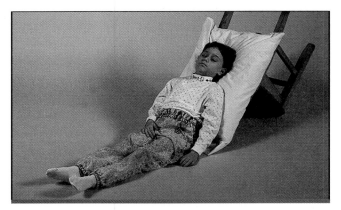

Raised head and shoulders position

Shock Position

Use this position if the child is exhibiting signs and symptoms of shock or if the seriousness of the injury causes you to think the child might go into shock. Lay the child flat on the back, using blankets or jackets to raise the feet 8 to 12 inches, but no more. This helps to increase the flow of blood to the heart and brain. Use this position only if you do not suspect a spine injury.

POSITIONING AN INJURED CHILD

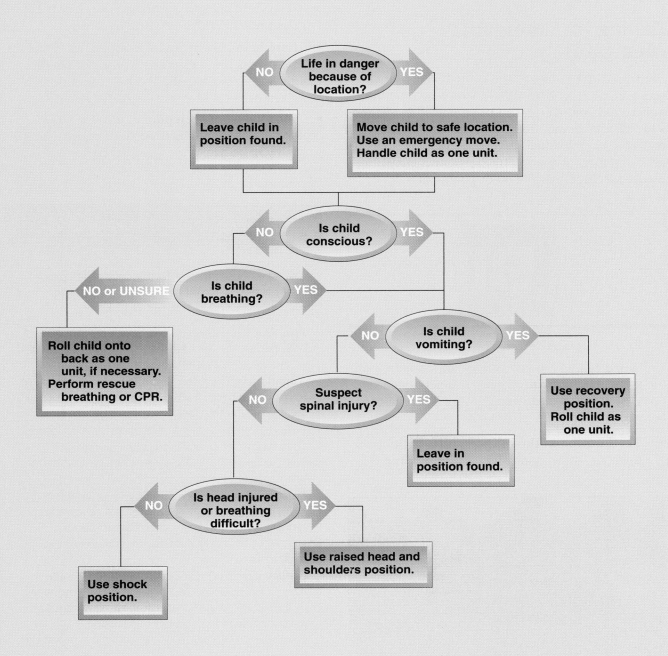

Life in danger because of location?

NO → **Leave child in position found.**

YES → **Move child to safe location. Use an emergency move. Handle child as one unit.**

Is child conscious?

NO → **Is child breathing?**

- NO or UNSURE → **Roll child onto back as one unit, if necessary. Perform rescue breathing or CPR.**
- YES →

YES → **Is child vomiting?**

- YES → **Use recovery position. Roll child as one unit.**
- NO → **Suspect spinal injury?**
  - YES → **Leave in position found.**
  - NO → **Is head injured or breathing difficult?**
    - YES → **Use raised head and shoulders position.**
    - NO → **Use shock position.**

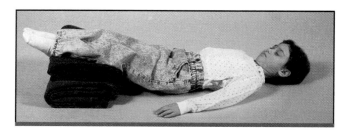

Shock position

Calling for Emergency Medical Help

In many communities in the United States, emergency medical services (EMS), which include fire, police, and ambulance, can be contacted by dialing 911. In other communities calls must be made directly to the individual services. Generally, emergency medical help is supplied by emergency medical technicians (EMTs) or paramedics.

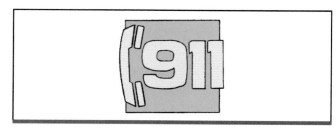

When calling for emergency medical help, give the following information over the telephone. Speak slowly and clearly and always be the last to hang up.

- **The location of the injured child.** Include the town and street name, house number, and the

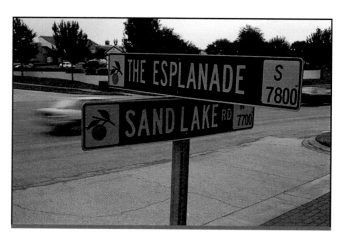

Crossed road signs

nearest intersecting street. Be specific in describing the building. If possible, send someone out to meet the ambulance. Ambulance drivers can waste precious minutes searching for an injured child because directions are not complete and street signs and numbers are not present or easily seen.

- **What happened.** Tell the dispatcher as much as you know. Explain what happened, such as, "The child fell and is unresponsive," or "The child has a cut that is bleeding heavily."

- **Care being given.** Tell the dispatcher what first aid care is being given to the injured child. The dispatcher can explain if other care should be given before emergency help arrives.

- **Your name and telephone number.** If additional information is needed, the dispatcher can call you back.

Emergency Telephone Numbers

The telephone numbers for the following emergency services should be posted by every telephone in your child care center or home.

Fire. Many fire departments have a rescue squad with paramedics or EMTs who respond quickly in an emergency situation.

Ambulance. The safest and often the fastest way to transport an injured child to an emergency medical facility is by ambulance.

Police. If necessary, police can transport an injured child to an emergency medical facility quickly. Many police officers are trained in CPR and rescue breathing.

Poison control center. Check your telephone book for the regional poison control center that serves your area. These centers are important sources of help and information and are available on a 24-hour basis.

Child's parent(s). Child care providers should have both the home and work telephone numbers of the child's parent(s). In addition, they should have the telephone number of a trusted neighbor or relative to contact if they are unable to reach the child's parent(s).

Child's health care provider. The child's health care provider should always be notified in an emergency.

If an injury occurs to a child in your child care setting, it is important to document the nature of the injury and the care provided. This information should be kept on file in the child care center. The injury report form below is provided as a sample of a document that can help the child care provider to adequately document the injury.

INJURY REPORT FORM

Child's name: _____ Birth date: _____

Date and time of injury: _____

Place where injury occurred: _____

Description of injury: _____

_____

_____

Description of how injury occurred: _____

_____

_____

Description of first aid care given: _____

_____

_____

First aid care given by: _____

Was EMS notified? _____

Was child's health care provider notified? _____

Adult witnesses to the injury: _____

_____

_____

Staff member supervising child at the time of the injury: _____

Child's parent notified: _____   _____

          Date   Time

_____   _____

Signature of person preparing this form   Date

Name _____ Course _____ Date _____

1. Fill in the blanks with the correct answers. In first aid, the letters "ABCD" stand for:

   A _airway_____

   B _Breathing_____

   C _Circulation_____

   D _CTS_____

2. Circle true (T) or false (F) for each statement about checking an injured child.

   (T) F   a. Never remove a child's medical alert tag.

   T   (F) b. A sign is a condition that the child feels.

   T   F   c. Healthy mucous membranes are moist and pink.

   (T) F   d. Changing an injured child's position could make a spine injury worse.

   (T) F   e. Most injuries require a complete head-to-toe examination.

3. Check the best answer. Before approaching a scene in which a child might be injured, your first step should be to:

   ____ a. Call the child's parent.

   ____ b. Determine if the injured child is unresponsive.

   ____ c. Make sure that it is safe for you to approach.

   ____ d. Perform the primary survey.

4. Match each position with its correct use after a traumatic injury.
   Raised head and shoulders position
   Recovery position
   Shock position

   a. _____ This side-lying position stabilizes the body, prevents the child from rolling forward or backward, and keeps the airway open.

   b. _____ This position helps to increase the flow of blood to the heart and brain.

   c. _____ This position makes breathing easier.

5. When calling for emergency medical help for a child, what information does the dispatcher need to know?

   a. _____

   b. _____

   c. _____

   d. _____

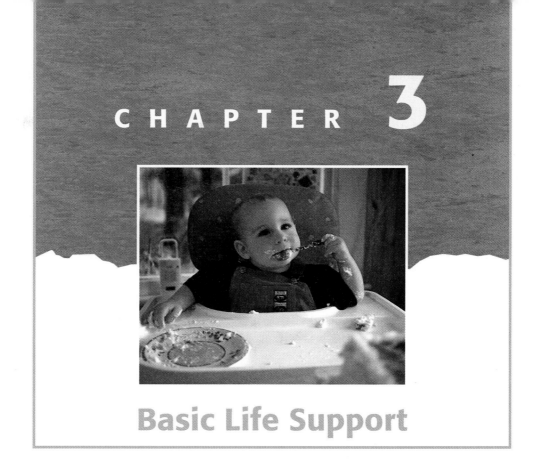

CHAPTER 3

Basic Life Support

This chapter provides an overview of CPR, rescue breathing, and related first aid issues for infants and children.

About CPR

Providing basic life support is the most important contribution you can make to another person's welfare. Rhythmic and uninterrupted breathing and a beating heart are essential for sustaining life. They are so intimately connected that if one stops, the other also stops.

The first aid provided when the vital functions of breathing and heartbeat stop is known as cardiopulmonary resuscitation, or CPR. *Cardio* refers to the heart and *pulmonary* refers to the lungs.

When the heart stops, all body functions, including breathing, also stop. CPR is a technique that combines breathing into another person's lungs with chest compressions on the breastbone, or sternum, to reproduce the work of the heart and lungs. CPR keeps oxygenated blood circulating to the vital organs—the heart, lungs, and brain.

Another technique, known as rescue breathing, is necessary when only the breathing stops. When breathing stops, the heart continues to beat for a few minutes. But without a continued supply of oxygen, the heart stops too. If rescue breathing is started immediately after breathing stops, there is a good chance of preventing the heart from stopping. A bystander can perform either rescue breathing or CPR, keeping oxygenated blood circulating to the vital organs while waiting for emergency medical help to arrive.

CPR is best learned in a classroom where you can practice the techniques on a mannikin and familiarize yourself with the process. Never practice any of these techniques on another person.

Please review the ABCDs in Chapter 2.

Who Needs CPR?

The health problems that first come to mind when we think about the need for CPR are heart attacks and strokes. Middle-aged and elderly adults who experience sudden death from some form of heart or artery disease are clearly the largest group for whom CPR techniques are intended.

But what about children? For most children, the heart is a healthy, strong muscle pumping blood through unobstructed blood vessels. When a healthy child's heart stops beating, it is seldom caused by a problem within the heart. Instead, the reason is likely an injury that causes the breathing to stop first. Some injuries that cause a child's breathing to stop are: electrocution, near-drowning, poisoning, smoke inhalation, severe trauma or head injury, and choking.

The Heart, Lung, and Brain Connection

All body tissues need oxygen to live. Oxygen enters the body through the lungs, where it passes into the blood. The heart then circulates this oxygen-rich blood to every cell in the body. The heart is a muscle about the size of your fist and is located in the center of the chest behind the sternum. The lungs lie on either side of the heart. Both heart and lungs are protected by the rib cage.

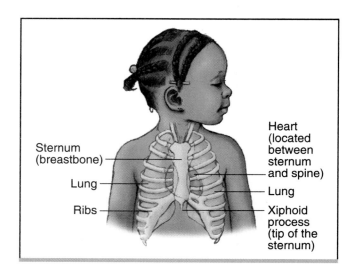

Location of heart and lungs

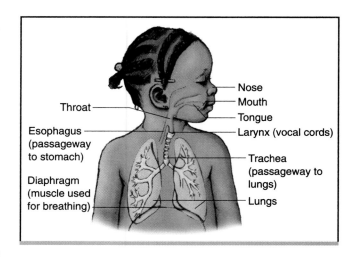

The respiratory system

The most demanding user of oxygen is the brain, the master control center of the body. This single organ needs about 20% of the total amount of oxygen used by the entire body. More significantly, the brain can survive without oxygen for only 4 to 6 minutes before the risk of brain damage becomes probable. The heart, too, can be damaged if it does not receive oxygen. This is why a *respiratory arrest* (when breathing stops) and a *cardiac arrest* (when the heart stops) are the most urgent life-threatening emergencies.

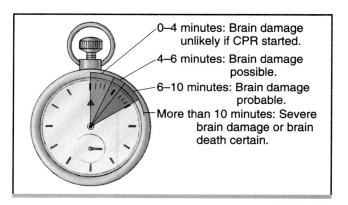

0–4 minutes: Brain damage unlikely if CPR started.
4–6 minutes: Brain damage possible.
6–10 minutes: Brain damage probable.
More than 10 minutes: Severe brain damage or brain death certain.

CPR can circulate enough oxygen to keep the brain and heart functioning. The air we inhale contains 21% oxygen. The body uses the oxygen it needs and then exhales air that contains 16% oxygen. This is why breathing into another person's lungs can provide that person with enough oxygen to keep the heart, lungs, and brain functioning.

The regular beating of the healthy heart pumps blood throughout the body with high efficiency. When the heart stops beating, external compression of the heart through CPR can restore 25% to 30%

of the normal blood circulation. In a crisis, the body naturally concentrates the available circulation to the most vital organs. So, even though CPR is not as efficient as normal breathing and circulation, it can be sufficient enough to sustain vital organs in an emergency. In the event of cardiac and respiratory arrest, the promptness with which CPR is started can determine the quality of life that will be enjoyed by the ill or injured person after recovery.

CPR Mouth Barriers

Current practice now includes using an infant-size or child-size CPR shield, mask, or other mouth barrier with a one-way valve. These barriers should be part of the first aid kit for use in a respiratory or cardiac emergency.

Keeping a Heart Healthy

The #1 killer of Americans is heart disease. Although heart disease is usually seen in adults, routine blood cholesterol screening of grade school children shows that, for some, high blood cholesterol levels are already present. These high cholesterol levels are known to contribute to heart disease. For many, lifestyle changes, such as diet and exercise, can reduce these levels and reduce the chance of developing heart disease later in life.

Both parents and child care providers are in a position to influence the behaviors, attitudes, and habits of young children in a positive way. Be a good role model and teach these heart-healthy habits:

- *Teach children not to smoke.* If you smoke, avoid doing so in front of children or in an area that will cause children and other staff to breathe the smoke. Both smokers and non-smokers should be aware of the dangers of smoking. Teach children that it is unhealthy to smoke ciagarettes. Consider stopping smoking for yourself and for the people who love you.
- *Teach children to eat healthy foods.* A lifetime of poor dietary habits can contribute to heart disease, especially diets that are high in fat. Children need to eat a variety of foods including cereals, breads, pasta, vegetables, fruits, low-fat dairy products, poultry, fish, and lean meats. Fats and sweets, although enjoyable, should be eaten sparingly. Talk about healthy foods at mealtimes and compliment the good choices that children make. If you eat with the children, be sure your meal is heart-healthy.
- *Teach children to exercise.* Most young children enjoy physical activity. Those who remain physically active over the years will reap the benefits as adults. Teach children that activities like running, swimming, outdoor games, riding bi-

cycles, and even jumping rope keep their heart muscles strong and healthy.

School-age children and adolescents need to learn about the additional factors of keeping both blood pressure and weight under control.

Call your local chapters of the American Heart Association and American Lung Association to learn about their educational materials for young children.

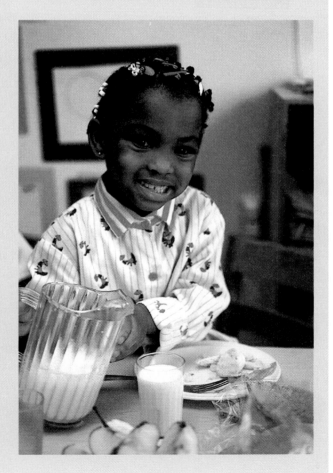

If you see a motionless child . . .

1

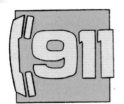

Check responsiveness

- Gently tap child's shoulder or back.
- Shout child's name and ask, "Are you okay?"
- If spine injury is suspected, move child only if absolutely necessary and avoid any twisting motion.

If child responds

Stop numbered rescue steps and check for other injuries.

2

Send someone to call for emergency medical help/emergency medical services (EMS)

If alone, shout for help and perform rescue breathing or CPR for 1 minute before making a telephone call yourself.

3

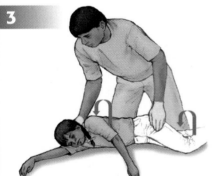

Roll child onto back

Avoid any twisting motion by taking the following steps:

- Straighten child's legs, if necessary.
- Move child's arm closest to you above child's head.
- Place one hand on child's neck and other hand on child's hip.
- Gently roll child toward you as one unit onto back.
- Place child's arms alongside body.

4

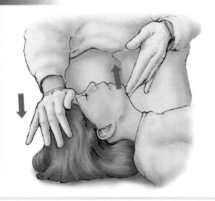

Open airway (use head-tilt/chin-lift method)

- Place hand nearest child's head on child's forehead and apply pressure to tilt head back to an above-neutral position.
- Place index and middle fingers of the other hand under bony part of jaw near chin and lift. Avoid pressing on soft tissue under jaw.
- Do not close child's mouth when tilting head.

4 **Continued**

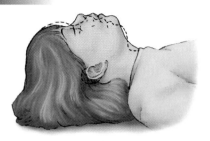

Drawing shows head in above-neutral position. Dashed line indicates neutral position.

If neck or spine injury is suspected

Open airway by lifting chin only. If this fails, tilt head backwards slightly until breath goes in. This is unlikely to further damage a spine injury.

If you see vomit

Wipe it out with gloved fingers or fingers covered by a cloth.

5

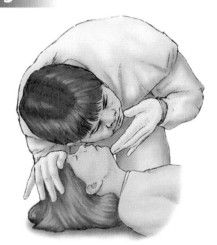

Check for breathing (take 3–5 seconds)

- Place your ear over child's mouth and nose while keeping airway open.
- *Look* for child's chest to rise and fall.
- *Listen* for breathing.
- *Feel* for breath against your cheek.

If child is breathing

Call for EMS if you have not already done so. Keep airway open and monitor breathing until EMS arrives.

6

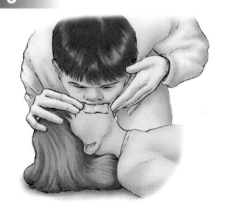

Give 2 slow breaths

- Keep airway open in an above-neutral position.
- Pinch child's nose shut.
- Make a seal around child's mouth with your mouth.
- Give 2 slow breaths, each lasting 1 to 1½ seconds. (Use a CPR mouth barrier if available.)
- Give breaths with just enough force for the child's chest to rise. You should be able to see this.
- Remove your mouth from child's after each breath to allow for chest deflation.

6 **Continued**

If first breath does not go in

Retilt child's head further back and try another breath. If second breath does not go in, suspect choking, also known as foreign-body airway obstruction. See *Unconscious Choking Child*.

If you are unable to make a seal around the child's mouth because of injury

Press against chin to close mouth, make a seal around nose, and breathe through nose.

7

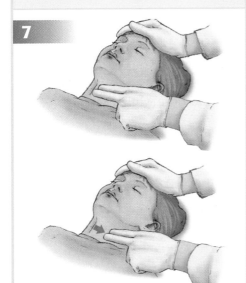

Check for pulse (take 5–10 seconds)

- Keep hand on child's forehead to maintain head tilt in an above-neutral position.
- Use index and middle fingers to locate Adam's apple with hand nearest child's feet.
- Slide your fingers down into groove of neck on side closest to you.
- Feel for carotid pulse.
- Do not use thumb to feel for pulse, because it has a pulse of its own.

8

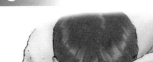

Perform rescue breathing or CPR based on what you find:

If there is a pulse but no breathing, begin rescue breathing

Maintain open airway with head-tilt/chin-lift. Pinch child's nose shut and make a seal around child's mouth with your mouth. Give one breath every 3 seconds. To do this, count: "one one-thousand," take a breath on "two one-thousand," and breathe into child on "three one-thousand." Give breaths with just enough force to see the child's chest rise. Remove your mouth after each breath to allow for chest deflation.

Pause to recheck pulse and breathing after each minute of rescue breathing (approximately 20 breaths). If alone, call for EMS now. Continue rescue breathing until:

- Child begins to breathe.
- A trained rescuer or EMS arrives to relieve you.
- You are too exhausted to continue rescue breathing.
- Injury scene becomes unsafe.

8 **Continued**

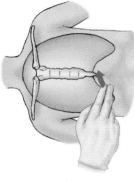

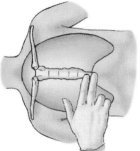

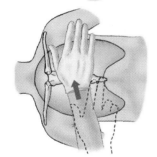

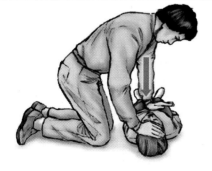

If there is no pulse or breathing, begin CPR

- Find compression location.

  1. Keep one hand on child's forehead to maintain head tilt.

  2. Slide fingers of other hand along edge of rib cage to notch at end of sternum.

  3. Cover notch with your middle finger and place your index finger beside it. Do not press on this notch.

  4. Remember location of index finger while you remove hand, and place heel of that hand on sternum next to index finger's prior location.

  5. Fingers should point across child's chest and away from you.

  6. Keep fingers off child's chest and keep elbow straight.

- Give 5 chest compressions.

  1. Give five compressions at a rate of 100 per minute, or 5 compressions in about 3 seconds. Count as you push down: "One, two, three, four, five."

  2. Compress sternum 1 to 1½ inches.

  3. Deliver compressions smoothly and rhythmically. Compression time should equal relaxation time. Blood is forced out of heart during compressions, and it flows into heart during relaxation, or when pressure is released.

  4. Keep heel of hand in contact with child's chest between compressions.

  5. Keep one hand on child's forehead to maintain head tilt.

8 **Continued**

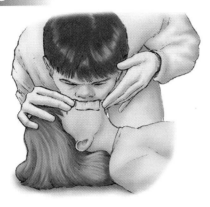

- Give 1 breath.

  1. Use head-tilt/chin-lift to keep airway open in an above-neutral position.

  2. Pinch child's nose shut.

  3. Make a seal around child's mouth with your mouth.

  4. Give one slow breath lasting 1 to 1½ seconds with just enough force to see child's chest rise.

  5. Allow for chest deflation after each breath.

- Give compressions and breaths in cycles of 5 compressions to 1 breath. Repeat for about 1 minute (12 cycles).

- Pause to recheck pulse and breathing after 1 minute of CPR and every few minutes thereafter. If alone, call for EMS now.

If child has pulse but is not breathing

Begin rescue breathing.

If child has no pulse

Continue CPR, beginning with chest compressions, until:

- Child has a pulse and is breathing.
- A trained rescuer or EMS arrives to relieve you.
- You are too exhausted to continue CPR.
- Scene becomes unsafe.

If there is more than one rescuer . . .

If you are performing CPR and another trained rescuer arrives to help

- Ask the other rescuer to determine if EMS has been called.
- Finish your compression/breathing cycle with a breath.
- The other rescuer checks the pulse for 5 seconds and continues CPR beginning with chest compressions.
- The other rescuer continues CPR until exhausted and asks you to take over again.
- The rescuer who is not performing CPR can check the effectiveness of the chest compressions by feeling for the carotid pulse during compressions.

Child (1–8 years) Rescue Breathing and CPR

If you arrive on a scene where a first rescuer is performing CPR

- Call EMS if it has not already been done.
- Tell the first rescuer that EMS has been called and that you know CPR and are able to help.

If a rescuer performing CPR asks you to take over

- Wait until the rescuer finishes a cycle of 5 chest compressions and one breath.
- Check the pulse for 5 seconds.
- If there is no pulse, continue CPR, beginning with chest compressions.

Conscious Choking Child (1–8 years)

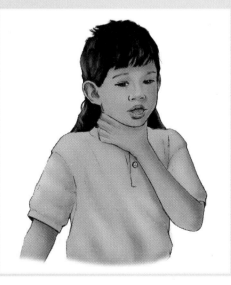

If child is coughing forcefully and you suspect that child has a foreign body (such as a piece of food or small toy part) caught in airway

Encourage child to continue coughing. Do not interfere with child's attempt to cough up object, do not slap child on back, and do not attempt abdominal thrusts.

If child is coughing weakly or cannot speak, cough, cry or breathe, assume child's airway is completely blocked

The child might also exhibit a panicked expression, make high-pitched noises in an effort to breathe, have blue lips and nails, and clutch at the throat, known as the "universal distress signal" for choking. Ask the child, "Can you speak?" If child cannot speak:

1

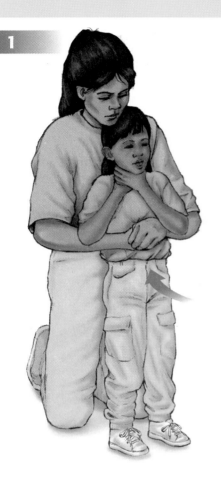

Give up to 5 abdominal thrusts (Heimlich maneuver)

- Stand or kneel behind child with your shoulders at about same level as child's.
- Wrap your arms around child's waist.
- Make a fist with one hand and place thumb side just above child's navel and well below tip of sternum.
- Grasp fist with your other hand.
- Press fist into child's abdomen with quick upward thrusts.
- Each thrust should be a separate and distinct effort to dislodge object.
- Keep fist in contact with abdomen between thrusts.

Pause after every series of 5 abdominal thrusts to check child and your hand placement.

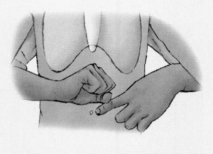

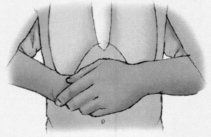

Hand placement for abdominal thrusts

2

Repeat cycles of up to 5 abdominal thrusts until:

- Child coughs up object.
- Child starts to breathe.
- Child becomes unconscious.
- A trained rescuer or EMS arrives to relieve you.

A child who has been given abdominal thrusts should be examined by a health care provider.

Unconscious Choking Child
(1–8 years)

If breaths have not gone in . . .

1

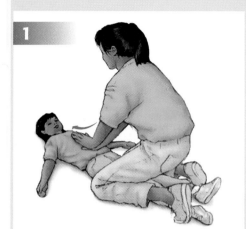

Give up to 5 abdominal thrusts (Heimlich maneuver)

- Kneel at child's feet or straddle child's thighs.
- Put heel of one hand against middle of child's abdomen, slightly above navel and well below notch at end of sternum.
- Place your other hand directly on top of first hand. Fingers should point toward child's head.
- Press inward and upward using both hands as a single unit, but allowing only heel of lower hand to touch abdomen. Keep heel of hand in contact with abdomen between abdominal thrusts.
- Give up to 5 abdominal thrusts. Deliver each thrust firmly and separately, as if each one will expel object.

2

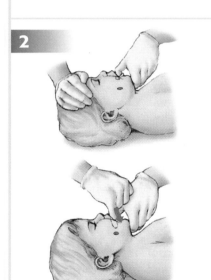

Check for foreign object

- Position yourself at child's head.
- Grasp both tongue and lower jaw between your thumb and fingers and lift jaw upward.
- Remove an object with a finger sweep only if you can see it: Slide the little finger of your free hand along inside of cheek to base of tongue, using a hooking action.
- Do not try to hook an object unless you can see it, because the attempt could push object deeper into airway.

3

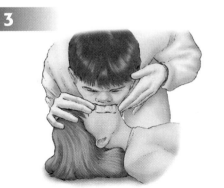

Give 1 breath

- Open airway with head-tilt/chin-lift.
- Pinch child's nose shut.
- Seal your mouth around child's mouth.
- Attempt to give 1 breath.

4

Repeat these steps until object is dislodged or expelled:

- Give up to 5 abdominal thrusts.
- Check for foreign object.
- Give one breath.

When object is expelled

Check pulse and breathing and treat accordingly.

Infant (up to 1 year) Rescue Breathing and CPR

If you find a motionless infant . . .

1

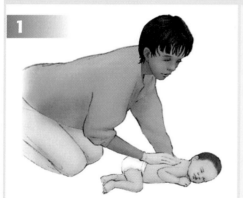

Check responsiveness

- Gently tap infant's shoulder or back.
- Call infant's name.
- If spine injury is suspected, move only if absolutely necessary and avoid any twisting motion.

If infant responds

Stop numbered rescue steps and check for other injuries

2

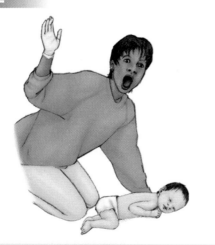

Send someone to call for emergency medical help/emergency medical services (EMS)

If alone, shout for help and perform rescue breathing or CPR for one minute before making a telephone call yourself.

3

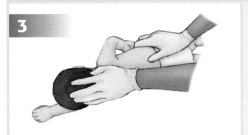

Roll infant onto back

Avoid any twisting motion by taking the following steps:

- Move infant's arm closest to you above infant's head.
- Place one hand on infant's neck and other hand on infant's hip.
- Gently roll infant toward you as one unit onto back.
- Place infant's arms alongside body. ·

4

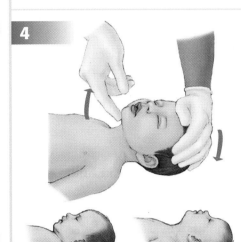

Too little tilt   Too much tilt

Open airway (use head-tilt/chin-lift method)

- Place hand nearest infant's head on infant's forehead and apply pressure to tilt head back slightly into a neutral position.
- Place index finger of other hand under bony part of jaw near chin and lift. Avoid pressing on soft tissue under jaw.
- Do not close infant's mouth when tilting head.

If neck or spinal injury is suspected

Open airway by lifting chin only. If this fails, tilt head backwards slightly until breath goes in. This is unlikely to further damage a spine injury.

If you see vomit

Wipe it out with gloved fingers or fingers covered by a cloth.

5

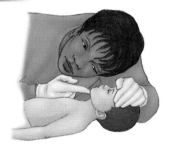

Check for breathing (take 3–5 seconds)

- Place your ear over infant's mouth and nose, while keeping the airway open.
- *Look* for infant's chest to rise and fall.
- *Listen* for breathing.
- *Feel* for breath against your cheek.

If infant is breathing

Call for EMS if not already done. Keep airway open and monitor breathing until EMS arrives.

6

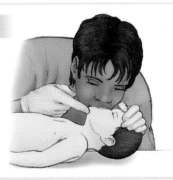

Give 2 slow breaths

- Use head-tilt/chin-lift to keep airway open in a neutral position.
- Make a seal around infant's nose and mouth with your mouth.
- Give 2 slow breaths, each lasting 1 to 1½ seconds. (Use a CPR mouth barrier if available.)
- Give breaths with just enough force to see infant's chest rise.
- Remove mouth after each breath to allow for chest deflation.

6 | **Continued**

If first breath does not go in

Retilt infant's head further back and try another breath. If second breath does not go in, suspect choking, also known as foreign-body airway obstruction. See *Unconscious Choking Infant*.

7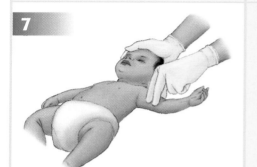

Check for pulse (take 5–10 seconds)

- Keep hand on infant's forehead to maintain head tilt in neutral position.
- Feel for brachial pulse on inside of upper arm between elbow and shoulder. Grip arm between fingers and thumb, using fingers to feel for pulse.
- Do not use your thumb to feel for pulse, because it has a pulse of its own.

8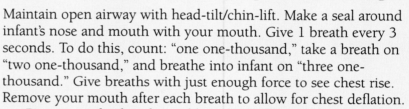

Perform rescue breathing or CPR based on what you find:

If there is a pulse but no breathing, begin rescue breathing

Maintain open airway with head-tilt/chin-lift. Make a seal around infant's nose and mouth with your mouth. Give 1 breath every 3 seconds. To do this, count: "one one-thousand," take a breath on "two one-thousand," and breathe into infant on "three one-thousand." Give breaths with just enough force to see chest rise. Remove your mouth after each breath to allow for chest deflation.

Pause to recheck pulse and breathing after each minute of rescue breathing (approximately 20 breaths). If alone, call for EMS now. Continue rescue breathing until:

- Infant begins to breathe.
- A trained rescuer or EMS arrives to relieve you.
- You are too exhausted to continue rescue breathing.
- Injury scene becomes unsafe.

If there is no pulse or breathing, begin CPR

- Find compression location.

  1. Keep one hand on infant's forehead to maintain head tilt.

  2. Imagine a line connecting the nipples.

  3. Place 3 fingers on sternum with index finger touching, but below imaginary nipple line.

  4. Lift your index finger and compress with middle and ring fingers. If you feel notch at end of sternum (xiphoid process), move your fingers up a little.

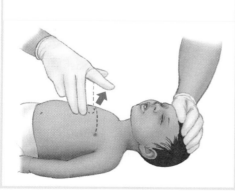

8 **Continued**

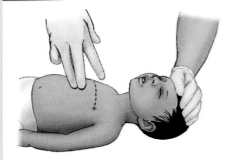

- Give 5 chest compressions.

  1. Give 5 compressions at a rate of at least 100 per minute, or 5 compressions in about 3 seconds. Count as you push down: "One, two, three, four, five."

  2. Compress sternum ½ to 1 inch.

  3. Deliver compressions smoothly and rhythmically. Compression time should equal relaxation time. Blood is forced out of heart during compressions and it flows into heart during relaxation, or when pressure is released.

  4. Keep tips of fingers in contact with infant's chest between compressions.

- Give 1 breath.

  1. Use head-tilt/chin-lift to keep airway open in a neutral position.

  2. Make a seal around infant's mouth and nose with your mouth.

  3. Give one breath lasting 1 to 1½ seconds with just enough force to see infant's chest rise.

  4. Allow for chest deflation after each breath.

- Give compressions and breaths in cycles of 5 compressions to 1 breath. Repeat for about 1 minute (20 cycles).

- Pause to recheck pulse and breathing after 1 minute of CPR and every few minutes thereafter. If alone, call for EMS now.

If infant has pulse, but is not breathing

Begin rescue breathing.

If infant has no pulse

Continue CPR, beginning with chest compressions, until:

- Infant has a pulse and is breathing.
- A trained rescuer or EMS arrives to relieve you.
- You are too exhausted to continue CPR.
- Injury scene becomes unsafe.

Conscious Choking Infant
(up to 1 year)

If an infant is coughing forcefully and you suspect that the infant has a foreign body (such as a piece of food or small toy part) caught in airway

Encourage infant to continue coughing. Place infant in upright position. Do not interfere with infant's attempt to cough up object, do not slap infant on back, and do not attempt chest thrusts.

If infant is coughing weakly or cannot cough, cry, or breathe, assume infant's airway is completely blocked.

The infant might also have blue lips and make high pitched noises in an effort to breathe.

1

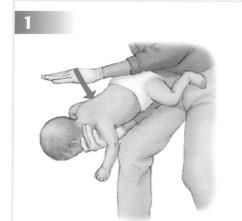

Give up to 5 back blows

- Lay infant face down along your forearm. Support infant's head and neck by holding jaw between your thumb and fingers with head lower than chest.
- Support your forearm against your thigh.
- Give up to 5 back blows between shoulder blades with heel of one hand.
- Deliver blows firmly and separately, as if each one will expel obstruction.

2

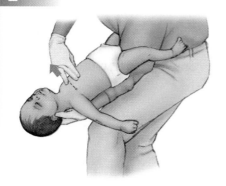

Give up to 5 chest thrusts

- Sandwich infant between your hands and forearms, and turn infant onto back with head lower than chest.
- Support back of infant's head and neck with your hand, and brace your forearm against your thigh.
- Just below an imaginary nipple line, place 3 fingers on sternum, or breastbone.
- Lift your ring finger off chest. If you feel notch at end of sternum (xiphoid process), move your fingers upward slightly.
- Give up to 5 chest thrusts by compressing sternum approximately ½ to 1 inch with index and middle fingers.
- Keep fingers in contact with chest between thrusts.

Conscious Choking Infant
(up to 1 year)

3

Repeat cycles of up to 5 back blows alternating with up to 5 chest thrusts until:

- Infant coughs up object.
- Infant starts to breathe.
- Infant becomes unconscious.
- A trained rescuer or EMS arrives to relieve you.

An infant who has been given back blows or chest thrusts should be examined by a health care provider.

Unconscious Choking Infant
(up to 1 year)

If breaths have not gone in . . .

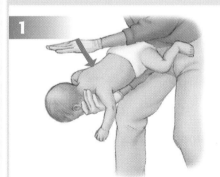

1

Give up to 5 back blows

- Lay infant face down along your forearm. Support infant's head and neck by holding jaw between your thumb and fingers with head lower than chest.
- Support your forearm against your thigh.
- Give up to 5 back blows between shoulder blades with heel of one hand.
- Deliver blows firmly and separately, as if each one will expel obstruction.

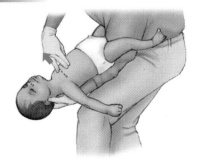

2

Give up to 5 chest thrusts

- Sandwich infant between your hands and forearms, and turn infant onto back with head lower than chest.
- Support back of infant's head and neck with your hand, and brace your forearm against your thigh.
- Just below an imaginary nipple line, place 3 fingers on sternum, or breast bone.
- Lift your ring finger off chest. If you feel notch at end of sternum (xiphoid process), move your fingers upward slightly.
- Give up to 5 chest thrusts by compressing sternum approximately ½ to 1 inch with index and middle fingers.
- Keep fingers in contact with chest between thrusts.
- Deliver each thrust firmly and separately, as if each one will expel obstruction.

3

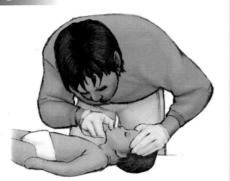

Check for foreign object

- Lay infant on floor or table, face up.
- Grasp tongue and lower jaw between your thumb and fingers and lift upward.
- Remove an object with a finger sweep only if you can see it: Slide the little finger of your free hand along the inside of cheek to base of tongue, using a hooking action.
- Do not try to hook an object unless you can see it, because the attempt could push object deeper into airway.

4

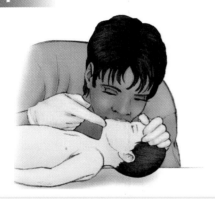

Give 1 breath

- Open airway using head-tilt/chin-lift.
- Seal your mouth around infant's mouth and nose.
- Attempt to give 1 breath.

5

Repeat these steps until object is dislodged or expelled:

- Give up to 5 back blows.
- Give up to 5 chest thrusts.
- Check for foreign object.
- Give 1 breath.

When object is expelled

Check pulse and breathing and treat accordingly.

Providing the Most Effective Chest Compressions

- Compress straight up and down in a smooth motion. Jerking and rocking back and forth reduce the force of the compression and can cause damage.
- Bend at the hips, not the waist, when compressing the child's chest.
- Keep the elbows locked and your shoulders positioned over the child's sternum.
- Do not compress the tip of the sternum. This soft cartilage notch (xiphoid process) can be injured and pushed into nearby tissues and organs.
- Keep the hand in contact with the chest between compressions; this will help to maintain correct hand position.
- When performing CPR on a child, allow only the heel of the hand, not the fingers, to come in contact with the chest.

Important Points in CPR Emergencies

- Because there is a risk of injury in performing CPR, no part of CPR should be performed on a child who does not need it. Be absolutely certain that the infant or child victim is unconscious and not just sleeping. Never practice CPR on a human being.
- An infant's airway is opened by tipping the head backward *slightly* into a neutral position. Overextending the backward tip of the head can reduce or even close the airway. A child's airway is opened by tipping the head back into an above-neutral position. The larger the child, the farther back the head must be tipped to open the airway.
- Touch only the bony part of the jaw near the chin when opening the airway. Do not touch the soft tissue of the throat.
- Opening the airway by tilting the head back moves the tongue out of the airway. In an unconscious person, the tongue is the most common airway obstruction.
- If injuries around the mouth prevent you from being able to make a tight seal, close the mouth by pushing against the chin and then breathe into the nose.
- Make sure that you use your fingers, not your thumb, to feel the carotid pulse, because your thumb has a pulse of its own.
- If you do not suspect a head or spine injury, carry the child to the telephone. This allows you to perform rescue breathing or CPR while calling for emergency medical help.
- A child who requires any basic life support technique should be examined in an emergency medical facility even if the child appears to have recovered fully.
- If the child who requires CPR is not revived within 1 minute, it is unlikely that CPR alone will revive the child. CPR, however, can keep the child's vital organs functioning until further emergency medical treatment can be started.

Complications of Performing CPR

Air in the Stomach

Sometimes air can be forced into a child's stomach when the rescuer is delivering breaths. This can reduce room for lung expansion and can lead to vomiting.

Air can be forced into the child's stomach by:

- Giving breaths too quickly
- Giving breaths too forcefully
- Not tilting the child's head back far enough

To keep air from being forced into the stomach while giving breaths:

- Allow enough time for the lungs to deflate between breaths
- Give only enough breath to see the chest rise
- Make certain that the child's head is tilted back far enough

If you notice that the child's stomach is beginning to appear bloated, do not attempt to remove the air by pressing on the stomach. Recheck your technique and continue breaths.

Vomiting

Because stomach contents contain acidic gastric juices, it can be especially dangerous if even a tiny amount enters the lungs. If a child or infant begins to vomit while you are performing CPR, immediately turn the head and body to one side to allow the vomitus to drain. Sweep the mouth clean, reposition the child or infant on the back, and continue CPR.

Compression Injuries

The actions necessary to perform CPR correctly require some degree of force. It is possible, although infrequent, in children that an injury to the ribs, lungs, or other organs can occur, despite correct CPR technique. Continue CPR even if you think a compression injury might have occurred. Such an injury can receive medical treatment later, but basic life support must not be interrupted.

Airway Obstruction Resulting from Illness

Occasionally in children, breathing difficulty leading to airway obstruction is caused by infection in the respiratory tract or by a severe allergic reaction. A child who is ill, with or without fever, and experiencing a barking cough and progressive difficulty breathing needs immediate care in an emergency medical facility.

The Heimlich maneuver and rescue breathing techniques will not help this child because the airway blockage is caused by swollen throat tissue, not a foreign object. Attempting these techniques can be dangerous and may postpone providing the care the child urgently needs. It is important to understand the difference between the sick child's emergency and the otherwise healthy child who suddenly begins to choke.

Basic Life Support Proficiency Checklist

S = self-check / P = partner check / I = instructor check

Child Rescue Breathing   S P I

1. Check responsiveness. ☐ ☐ ☐
2. Send someone to call EMS. ☐ ☐ ☐
3. Roll child onto back. ☐ ☐ ☐
4. Open airway (to above-neutral position). ☐ ☐ ☐
5. Check for breathing (take 3–5 sec.). ☐ ☐ ☐
6. Give 2 slow breaths (1 to 1½ sec. each). ☐ ☐ ☐
7. Check for carotid pulse (take 5–10 sec.). ☐ ☐ ☐
8. Perform rescue breathing (1 breath every 3 sec.). ☐ ☐ ☐
9. Recheck pulse and breathing after 20 breaths or about 1 min. ☐ ☐ ☐
10. Continue rescue breathing (rechecking pulse and breathing every 20 breaths or about 1 min.). ☐ ☐ ☐

Child CPR   S P I

1. Check responsiveness. ☐ ☐ ☐
2. Send someone to call EMS. ☐ ☐ ☐
3. Roll child onto back. ☐ ☐ ☐
4. Open airway (to above-neutral position). ☐ ☐ ☐
5. Check for breathing (take 3–5 sec.). ☐ ☐ ☐
6. Give 2 slow breaths 1 to 1½ sec. each). ☐ ☐ ☐
7. Check for carotid pulse (take 5–10 sec.). ☐ ☐ ☐
8. Find compression location. ☐ ☐ ☐

9. Perform CPR (5 compressions to 1 breath for 12 cycles or about 1 min.). ☐ ☐ ☐
10. Recheck pulse. ☐ ☐ ☐
11. Continue CPR (rechecking pulse every few min.). ☐ ☐ ☐

Conscious Choking Child   S P I

1. Determine if child is choking. ☐ ☐ ☐
2. Give up to 5 abdominal thrusts. ☐ ☐ ☐
3. Check child and check your hand position. ☐ ☐ ☐
4. Continue cycles of abdominal thrusts and checks. ☐ ☐ ☐

Unconscious Choking Child S P I

1. Check responsiveness. ☐ ☐ ☐
2. Send someone to call EMS. ☐ ☐ ☐
3. Roll child onto back. ☐ ☐ ☐
4. Open airway (to above-neutral position). ☐ ☐ ☐
5. Check for breathing (take 3–5 sec.). ☐ ☐ ☐
6. Attempt to give 2 slow breaths. ☐ ☐ ☐
7. If first breath unsuccessful, retilt head and try another breath. ☐ ☐ ☐
8. Give up to 5 abdominal thrusts. ☐ ☐ ☐
9. Check for foreign object. ☐ ☐ ☐
10. Attempt to give a breath. ☐ ☐ ☐
11. Repeat sequences of thrusts, check, and breath. ☐ ☐ ☐

Basic Life Support Proficiency Checklist

S = self-check / P = partner check / I = instructor check

Infant Rescue Breathing   S   P   I

1. Check responsiveness. ☐ ☐ ☐
2. Send someone to call EMS. ☐ ☐ ☐
3. Roll infant onto back. ☐ ☐ ☐
4. Open airway (to neutral position). ☐ ☐ ☐
5. Check for breathing (take 3–5 sec.). ☐ ☐ ☐
6. Give 2 slow breaths (1 to 1½ sec.). ☐ ☐ ☐
7. Check for brachial pulse (Take 5–10 sec.). ☐ ☐ ☐
8. Perform rescue breathing (1 breath every 3 sec.). ☐ ☐ ☐
9. Recheck pulse and breathing after 20 breaths or about 1 min. ☐ ☐ ☐
10. Continue rescue breathing (rechecking pulse and breathing every 20 breaths or about 1 min.). ☐ ☐ ☐

Infant CPR   S   P   I

1. Check responsiveness. ☐ ☐ ☐
2. Send someone to call EMS. ☐ ☐ ☐
3. Roll infant onto back. ☐ ☐ ☐
4. Open airway (to neutral position). ☐ ☐ ☐
5. Check for breathing (take 3–5 sec.). ☐ ☐ ☐
6. Give 2 slow breaths (1 to 1½ sec.). ☐ ☐ ☐
7. Check for brachial pulse (take 5–10 sec.). ☐ ☐ ☐
8. Find compression location. ☐ ☐ ☐
9. Perform CPR (5 compressions to 1 breath for 20 cycles or about 1 min.). ☐ ☐ ☐
10. Recheck pulse. ☐ ☐ ☐
11. Continue CPR (rechecking pulse every few min.). ☐ ☐ ☐

Conscious Choking Infant   S   P   I

1. Determine if infant is choking. ☐ ☐ ☐
2. Give up to 5 back blows and up to 5 chest thrusts. ☐ ☐ ☐
3. Continue cycles until successful or infant becomes unconscious. ☐ ☐ ☐

Unconscious Choking Infant   S   P   I

1. Check responsiveness. ☐ ☐ ☐
2. Send someone to call EMS. ☐ ☐ ☐
3. Roll infant onto back. ☐ ☐ ☐
4. Open airway (to neutral position). ☐ ☐ ☐
5. Check for breathing (take 3–5 sec.). ☐ ☐ ☐
6. Attempt to give 2 slow breaths. ☐ ☐ ☐
7. If first breath unsuccessful, retilt head and try another breath. ☐ ☐ ☐
8. Give up to 5 back blows. ☐ ☐ ☐
9. Give up to 5 chest thrusts. ☐ ☐ ☐
10. Check for foreign object. ☐ ☐ ☐

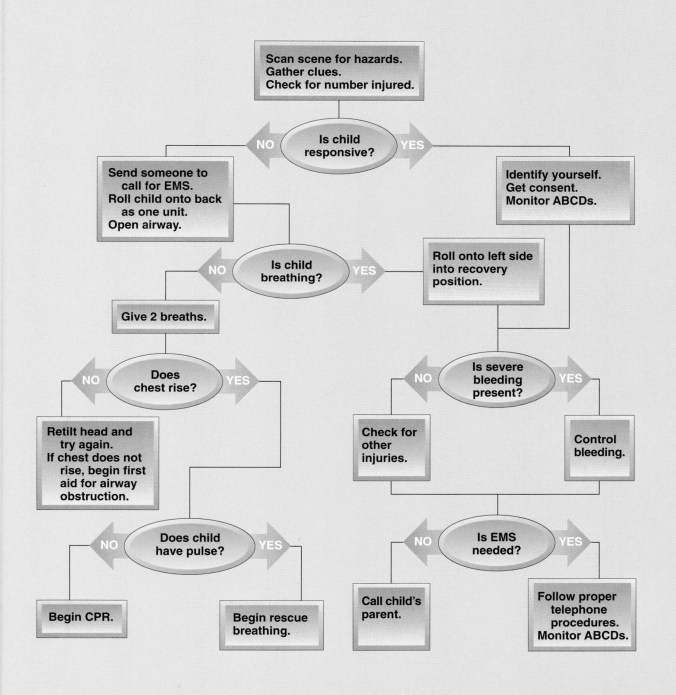

Name _____ Course _____ Date _____

1. Fill in the blank with the correct answer.
   a. When giving rescue breaths to a child, give 1 breath every _____ seconds.
   b. Compress an infant's chest _____ inch(es) when performing CPR.

2. Circle true (T) or false (F) for each question about CPR and rescue breathing.

   T   F   a. Chest compressions for a child should be given at a rate of 80 compressions per minute.

   T   F   b. The compression location for an infant is located well below the xiphoid notch.

   T   F   c. When giving rescue breaths to a child, give breath with just enough force to see the chest rise.

   T   F   d. When performing rescue breathing on a child, keep the airway open by tipping child's head forward in an above-neutral position.

   T   F   e. When giving chest compressions to an infant, use the heel of one hand.

   T   F   f. Perform chest compressions with a smooth rhythmic motion.

3. Check the correct answer. To determine if an unresponsive child has stopped breathing, you should:
   ___ a. Check for a pulse.
   ___ b. Look at the child's pupils.
   ___ c. Look, listen, and feel for breaths.

4. During lunch at your center, 3-year-old Julia laughs while eating, and suddenly she cannot speak or cough. You should:
   ___ a. Look in her mouth to determine the cause.
   ___ b. Slap her on the back several times until she coughs.

   ___ c. Encourage her to cough.
   ___ d. Give 5 abdominal thrusts.

5. Two-year-old Mario pulls a button from his overalls, puts it in his mouth, and chokes on it. He is conscious and coughing forcefully. You should:
   ___ a. Encourage him to continue coughing.
   ___ b. Give 5 back blows.
   ___ c. Check for a foreign object.
   ___ d. Give 5 abdominal thrusts.

6. You see a child lying on the ground at your local playground. She does not respond when you call to her. Your next step should be:
   ___ a. Open the airway.
   ___ b. Roll her onto the back and begin rescue breathing.
   ___ c. Send someone to call for emergency medical help.
   ___ d. Give five abdominal thrusts.

7. You open the airway of an unresponsive child. You try to give a breath, but the air does not go in. You reposition the head and try again, but the air will not go in. What should you do next?
   ___ a. Give up to 5 abdominal thrusts.
   ___ b. Check for a foreign object.
   ___ c. Reposition the head and try giving breaths again.
   ___ d. Give up to 5 back blows.

8. Eight-month-old Rae is choking on a piece of apple. She is conscious but cannot cough, cry, or breathe. You should:
   ___ a. Encourage her to cough.
   ___ b. Give up to 5 abdominal thrusts.
   ___ c. Give up to 5 back blows and up to 5 chest thrusts.
   ___ d. Check for a foreign object.

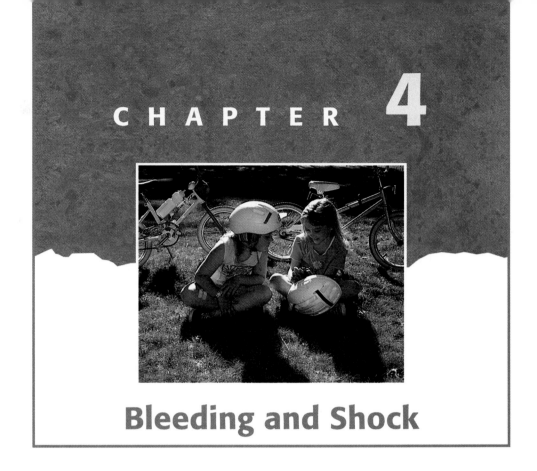

CHAPTER 4

Bleeding and Shock

When the skin is cut and a blood vessel of any size is broken, bleeding occurs. The seriousness of the injury is determined by how deep the cut is, the type of blood vessels damaged, the amount of bleeding that occurs, and the time it takes to control it.

The most severe bleeding is from arteries, which are large, deeply located, and well-protected blood vessels. Injury to an artery is, therefore, infrequent but serious when it occurs. Arteries carry blood away from the heart to all parts of the body under the strong pressure exerted by each heartbeat. Bright red arterial blood spurts from a damaged artery with each beat of the heart and can be difficult to control—even life-threatening.

Veins are blood vessels that carry blood back to the heart. They are located closer to the surface of the skin than arteries. Bleeding from veins is slower than from arteries because the blood is under less pressure. Although a vein can bleed heavily, it can usually be controlled with simple first aid measures. Venous blood is dark red in color.

Tiny blood vessels located throughout the body are called capillaries. There are hundreds of thousands of capillaries throughout the surface of the skin. When broken, their oozing is the most easily controlled.

Some parts of the body have more blood vessels than other parts do. For example, the head and face have an abundance of blood vessels, so a cut there bleeds profusely. The hands and feet have fewer blood vessels and a cut in these areas results in less blood loss.

We live in a time that makes wearing disposable gloves essential when giving first aid to someone else. Coming into contact with blood and other body fluids, such as stool, urine, mucus, and vomitus, can allow transmission of organisms such as the hepatitis B virus and HIV. These diseases threaten health and life. If disposable gloves are not immediately available, you should use another type of barrier. Have another person find your disposable gloves, while you use a thick protective barrier to begin first aid.

A protective barrier is a covering that provides a shield between your skin and another person's blood or other body fluids. Barriers also protect a child with an open wound from contaminants on your hands. Examples of protective barriers include:

- Disposable gloves
- A plastic bag or anything that is waterproof
- Several thick layers of gauze pads
- A thickly folded cloth diaper or dish towel

Plastic wrap placed over the gauze or cloth covering increases the effectiveness of these barriers. Keep a pair of disposable gloves in a handy and easily accessible location, such as your first aid kit, car glove compartment, fanny pack, or purse.

External Bleeding

Many children, as well as adults, become anxious at the sight of blood. In most situations, bleeding can be controlled in 5 to 10 minutes with proper first aid.

What to Do

1. Apply firm, direct pressure. Wear disposable gloves and cover the injury with several gauze pads or the cleanest covering available, such as a dish towel, and press firmly against it. Keep the pad or cloth in place for 5 to 10 minutes, without peeking. It is easier to see the extent of the injury after the bleeding has slowed or stopped. Direct pressure controls the bleeding at the injury, but it does not interrupt the blood flow to the uninjured surrounding areas.

2. Elevate the injured body part above the level of the heart without releasing the direct pressure. This uses gravity to slow the flow of blood.

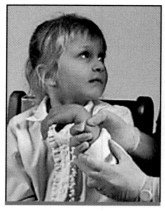
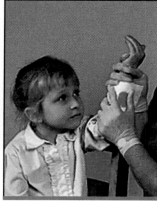

Apply firm, direct pressure.   Elevate without releasing direct pressure.

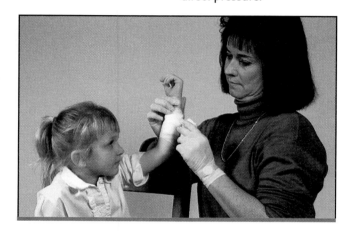

Apply a pressure bandage.

3. If necessary, maintain pressure by placing several gauze pads over the bleeding wound and securing them firmly with a roll of gauze or tape, making a *pressure bandage*. This keeps

DO NOT

- remove the original dressing. If it becomes soaked with blood, add another dressing.
- elevate an injured extremity if a fracture is suspected or if movement causes additional pain.
- attempt to apply a tourniquet and discourage others from doing so. A tourniquet cuts off the circulation to the entire injured limb and might make amputation necessary.
- release direct pressure on the wound when applying pressure on a pressure point.
- use direct pressure on a protruding bone, a skull fracture, an eye injury, or a wound with an embedded object.

pressure on the bleeding wound and frees your hands to attend to other injuries. Add more gauze pads or cloths on top of the original dressing if it becomes soaked with blood. Removing the original dressing disturbs the blood vessels and interferes with clotting. Clotting is the process that thickens the blood at the wound site to gradually stop the bleeding and seal the wound. In a small wound, this process takes 3 to 5 minutes to begin after the heavy flow of blood is reduced. For deep wounds, see *About Stitches.*

4. Apply pressure at a pressure point if severe bleeding cannot be controlled using direct pres-

sure and elevation. Continue to apply direct pressure on the wound. See *About Pressure Points.*

5. Treat for shock, if necessary. See *Shock.*

6. Call for emergency medical help, if necessary. Notify the child's parent.

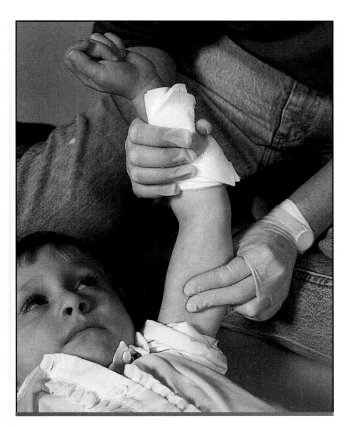

Apply pressure to the brachial pressure point.

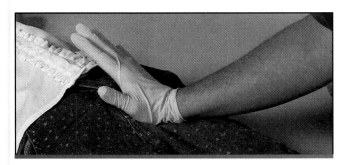

Apply pressure to the femoral pressure point.

About Pressure Points

Pressure points are used *only* when direct pressure and elevation alone cannot control severe bleeding or when direct pressure cannot be applied to a bleeding wound because of a protruding broken bone or an embedded object, such as a piece of glass.

A pressure point is located where a main artery passes over a bone between the injury and the heart. Compressing the artery against the bone slows the flow of blood to the bleeding limb. Because reducing blood flow to the entire arm or leg for a long period of time can cause irreparable damage to the limb, use pressure points *only* when necessary.

The pressure points used most often are the brachial and femoral pressure points, located on both sides of the body. Find the brachial pressure point by placing your fingertips inside the upper arm, halfway between the elbow and the underarm, in the groove between the muscles. Squeeze the arm firmly between the thumb and fingertips. Locate the femoral pressure point by placing the heel of your hand at the middle of the groin. Apply firm and steady pressure, but do not release direct pressure over the injury.

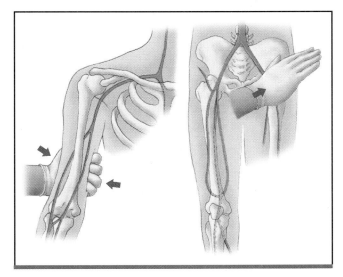

Brachial and femoral pressure point locations

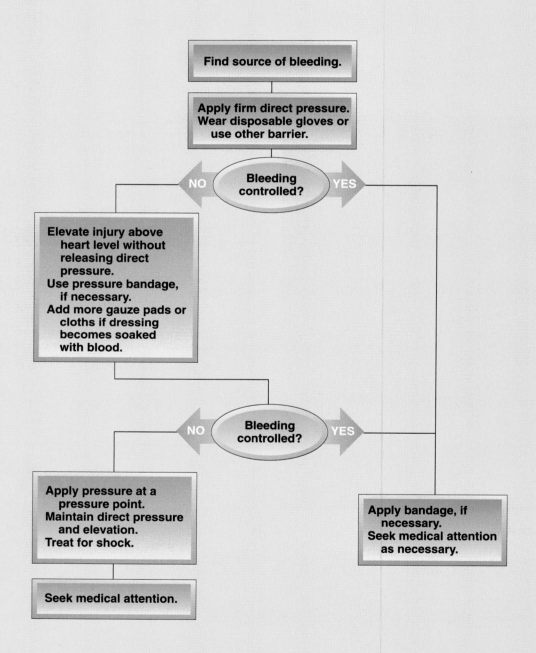

Find source of bleeding.

Apply firm direct pressure.
Wear disposable gloves or
use other barrier.

NO — **Bleeding controlled?** — YES

Elevate injury above
heart level without
releasing direct
pressure.
Use pressure bandage,
if necessary.
Add more gauze pads or
cloths if dressing
becomes soaked
with blood.

NO — **Bleeding controlled?** — YES

Apply pressure at a
pressure point.
Maintain direct pressure
and elevation.
Treat for shock.

Seek medical attention.

Apply bandage, if
necessary.
Seek medical attention
as necessary.

Internal Bleeding

Internal bleeding occurs when blood vessels inside the body are broken but the skin over the injury remains intact. Minor internal bleeding occurs when small capillaries are injured following a blow and results in bruising. Severe internal bleeding can result from a blunt abdominal injury forceful enough to damage large vessels or organs deep inside the chest or abdomen or from an injury that breaks a bone and punctures an internal structure, such as a broken rib puncturing a lung. Internal bleeding can also result from a medical problem such as a ruptured appendix. Severe internal bleeding is life-threatening.

What to Look For

- A scene suggesting that traumatic injury to the chest or abdomen has just occurred
- Vomiting or coughing up blood
- Painful, tender, rigid abdomen
- Large bruises on chest or abdomen

What to Do

1. Check the ABCDs and treat accordingly.
2. Send someone to call for emergency medical help.
3. Place the child on the left side in the recovery position to prevent choking if vomiting occurs.
4. Cover the child with a blanket or jacket to prevent heat loss but not to create additional warmth. Allowing a child to become too warm draws the blood to the skin and away from the vital organs. Place a blanket under the child's body to insulate the child from the ground and from further heat loss.

DO NOT
- give anything to eat or drink

Shock

Shock is the body's response to a disruption somewhere in the circulatory system that prevents blood from circulating in adequate amounts to all parts of the body, especially to the vital organs. Damage to the heart or blood vessels or a decrease in the amount of blood flow can cause shock.

Hypovolemic Shock

The most common form of shock in children is hypovolemic shock. It occurs when there is blood loss from either an obvious external wound or from a bleeding wound hidden deep inside the body. Shock can be life-threatening and occurs in the types of injuries sustained in a serious motor vehicle accident, bicycle accident, or fall. In adults, shock accompanies heart attacks and strokes.

Some degree of shock occurs with all injuries. With minor injuries, the body is able to recover on its own. With more serious injuries, the body cannot recover on its own, and death can result if emergency medical care is not provided.

Shock is most likely to occur within the first few minutes, but it can appear up to 2 hours after an injury. Treating for shock, whether or not signs and symptoms are present, is the safest way to proceed when caring for a child who has a serious injury. A first aider can slow the progress of shock and even prevent it from occurring by taking the correct steps immediately. Regardless of the cause, the signs and symptoms of shock and the first aid given are always the same.

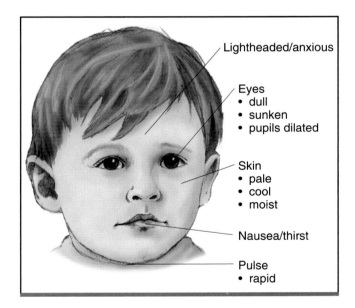

Signs and symptoms of shock

What to Look For

- Pale skin color. A blue or gray discoloration around the nose and mouth and a blue discoloring of the nailbeds shows that too little blood and oxygen are reaching these parts of the body.

- Cool, moist skin. The blood is concentrated in the vital organs deep inside the body and not in the blood vessels on the surface.
- Rapid, weak pulse. The heart is trying to compensate for the reduced amount of circulating blood and oxygen by beating faster.
- Rapid, shallow breathing
- Lightheadedness, anxiety, restlessness. The brain is not getting enough oxygen.
- Thirst
- Nausea

What to Do

1. Check the ABCDs, and use direct pressure, elevation, and pressure points to control severe bleeding.
2. Send someone to call for emergency medical help.
3. Place the child in the shock position by laying the child flat on the back and using blankets or jackets to raise the feet 8 to 12 inches but no more. This helps to increase the flow of blood to the heart and brain. If the child becomes unconscious or begins to vomit, place the child on the left side in the recovery position.
4. Cover the child with a blanket or jacket to prevent heat loss but not to create additional warmth. Allowing a child to become too warm draws the blood to the skin and away from the vital organs. Place a blanket under the child's body to insulate the child from the ground and from further heat loss.
5. Check for other injuries and treat accordingly. Shock always occurs in response to an injury; it does not happen on its own.

DO NOT

- **raise the legs any higher than 8 to 12 inches, because it will affect the child's breathing by pushing the abdominal organs against the diaphragm.**
- **give anything to eat or drink.**
- **raise the legs of a child with a suspected spine injury.**
- **raise the legs of a child with a head injury or with breathing difficulties.**

Anaphylaxis

Children who have allergies to such common agents as pollen, molds, dust, animal dander, or certain foods learn that avoidance is the best way to prevent the unpleasant reaction that their bodies produce. Most common allergic reactions can be brought under control by removing the cause from the child's environment or diet.

An uncommon and far more serious allergic reaction is known as anaphylaxis, which can be fatal if not reversed within minutes. It occurs suddenly, usually within seconds or minutes after coming in contact with the allergen. It causes many allergic symptoms, the most dangerous of which is swelling of the airway that cuts off the child's ability to breathe. If epinephrine, the medication that counteracts anaphylaxis, is not available, death can occur within minutes.

Anaphylaxis is unexpected because, initially, neither the child nor parent is aware of the child's extreme allergy to a substance that is harmless to most people. Anaphylaxis can occur in a child who receives a dose of a medication, such as penicillin or tetanus antitoxin, or after eating a food, such as shellfish, nuts, or eggs. A child might also eat a prepared food without knowing that it contains a food additive or ingredient to which the child is highly allergic. Stings from an insect of the Hymenoptera order, which includes bees, wasps, hornets, yellow jackets, and ants, can also cause anaphylaxis. See *Insect Stings*, Chapter 10. This allergy can develop at any time in life, no matter how many nonallergic stings a child has already had.

A child must be exposed to the allergen at least once in order for this extreme sensitivity to develop. The first exposure does not cause an allergic reaction. It does, however, cause excessive amounts of an antibody named immunoglobulin E (IgE) to be produced in the blood. When the allergen next enters the body and comes in contact with the IgE antibody, a series of dangerous internal reactions begin, which are known collectively as anaphylaxis. If this allergic reaction is severe, and if epinephrine, the medication that counteracts the anaphylaxis, is not available, anaphylactic shock and death can occur within minutes.

What to Look For

- Flushed skin
- Hives—a generalized rash of itchy, red, raised, blotchy areas on the skin

HYPOVOLEMIC SHOCK

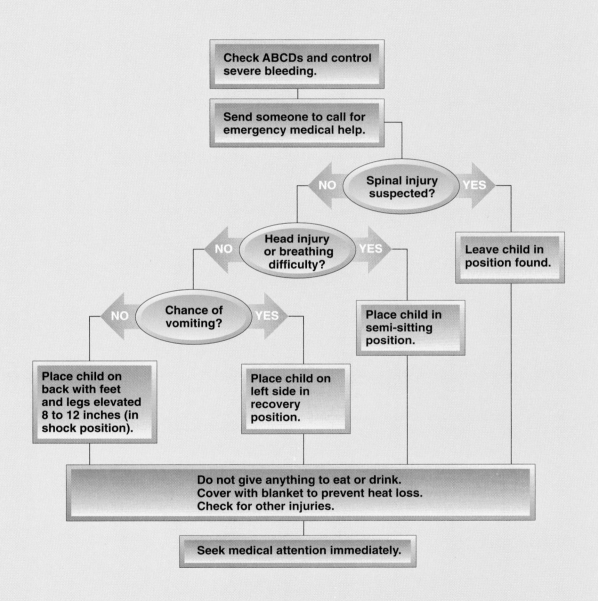

Check ABCDs and control severe bleeding.

Send someone to call for emergency medical help.

Spinal injury suspected?
- NO
- YES → Leave child in position found.

Head injury or breathing difficulty?
- NO
- YES → Place child in semi-sitting position.

Chance of vomiting?
- NO → Place child on back with feet and legs elevated 8 to 12 inches (in shock position).
- YES → Place child on left side in recovery position.

Do not give anything to eat or drink.
Cover with blanket to prevent heat loss.
Check for other injuries.

Seek medical attention immediately.

- Sudden uneasiness and anxiety
- Dizziness
- Swelling of the face, lips, and tongue; difficulty swallowing
- Abdominal or stomach cramps and diarrhea
- Wheezing or difficulty breathing because of swelling in the throat
- Tightness in the chest
- Bluish or grayish skin color around the lips and mouth
- Loss of consciousness
- Cardiovascular collapse—a heartbeat so weak that blood cannot circulate

What to Do

1. Send someone to call for emergency medical help.
2. Place an unresponsive child on the left side in the recovery position. Place a conscious child who is having trouble breathing in a sitting position to make breathing easier.
3. Administer epinephrine immediately. Epinephrine can be given by a parent or a child care provider who has been shown how to administer the medication. More than one dose of epinephrine is often necessary to reverse anaphylaxis.

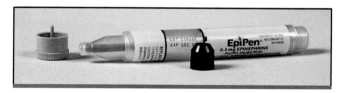

Allergic emergency kit

4. Monitor the ABCDs and treat accordingly. Rescue breathing is difficult and may be impossible because the child's airway is narrowed by the swelling.
5. Have the child seen immediately in an emergency medical facility. This is a life-threatening emergency!

Children who have had an extreme reaction to a specific allergen should have an allergic emergency kit (also known as an anaphylaxis kit or insect sting kit) containing the epinephrine injection. It should be stored with the first aid supplies in the child care center at room temperature. This is not a routine item in all first aid kits; it is a prescription drug intended specifically for the allergic child in an emergency. It contains an easy-to-use mechanism that administers the correct dose of the drug. At least one staff member in a child care center should be taught how to use the kit. A school-aged child who has been given a kit by a pediatrician should always carry it.

Sometimes the signs and symptoms of an allergic reaction develop slowly over a period of 1 to 2 hours. The child should be taken to an emergency medical facility as soon as the reaction is recognized as such.

If the child experiences an allergic reaction, it is necessary to identify the allergen to prevent a second reaction that could be more severe. This child should always wear a medical alert necklace or bracelet that identifies the allergen. These products are available through many drugstores. As an additional precaution, parents might be advised to remain in the health care provider's office or the hospital for at least 30 minutes after their child receives a medication known to have the potential to cause an allergic reaction.

ANAPHYLAXIS

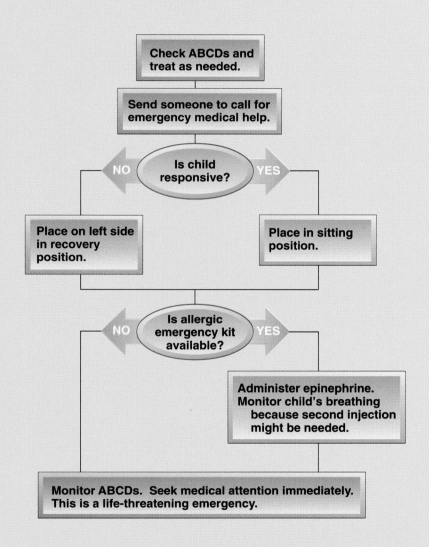

Check ABCDs and treat as needed.

Send someone to call for emergency medical help.

Is child responsive?

NO → Place on left side in recovery position.

YES → Place in sitting position.

Is allergic emergency kit available?

YES → Administer epinephrine. Monitor child's breathing because second injection might be needed.

NO → Monitor ABCDs. Seek medical attention immediately. This is a life-threatening emergency.

Name _____ Course _____ Date _____

1. Circle true (T) or false (F) for each statement about bleeding.

    T F a. The amount of bleeding from a wound depends, in part, on the type of blood vessels damaged.

    T F b. Bleeding from veins spurts and may be difficult to control.

    T F c. Arterial bleeding is usually more serious than venous bleeding.

    T F d. A first aider should wear disposable gloves when caring for a bleeding wound.

2. Circle yes (Y) or no (N) for each of the following statements. Which of the following action(s) should you use to control severe bleeding?

    Y N a. Place firm, direct pressure on the wound.

    Y N b. Release direct pressure if the arm is elevated.

    Y N c. Use a pressure point alone if direct pressure fails to stop the bleeding.

    Y N d. Replace a blood-soaked dressing with a clean dressing.

3. Circle true (T) or false (F) for each of the following statements about shock.

    T F a. Shock results when vital organs do not receive sufficient blood.

    T F b. Shock can occur several days after an injury.

    T F c. The most common form of shock in children is anaphylaxis.

    T F d. An injured child can breathe more easily in a semi-sitting position than in a lying-down position.

4. Circle true (T) or false (F) for each statement. When a child experiences hypovolemic shock, the:

    T F a. Skin is flushed.

    T F b. Skin is moist.

    T F c. Child feels thirsty.

    T F d. Breathing and pulse are rapid.

    T F e. Child feels hungry.

5. Circle yes (Y) or no (N) for each of the following actions concerning first aid for hypovolemic shock. A child begins to show signs of shock after an injury. Which of the following actions would you take?

    Y N a. Give fluids to the child.

    Y N b. Encourage the child to walk around to increase blood flow to the heart.

    Y N c. For difficulty breathing, place the child in a semi-sitting position.

    Y N d. Use several blankets or jackets to create additional warmth.

6. Give three signs or symptoms of anaphylaxis in a child.

    a. _____

    b. _____

    c. _____

7. Give three examples of what might cause a child to experience anaphylaxis.

    a. _____

    b. _____

    c. _____

8. Circle true (T) or false (F) for each the following questions about allergic reactions.

    T F a. Hives are a sign of an allergic reaction.

    T F b. A child experiencing anaphylaxis needs sugar immediately.

    T F c. The only effective treatment for anaphylaxis is epinephrine.

    T F d. Epinephrine is administered as an injection.

    T F e. Some allergic reactions can be severe enough to require CPR.

    T F f. Epinephrine is only available with a physician's prescription.

    T F g. Common agents, such as pollen, molds, and dust, can cause anaphylaxis.

    T F h. More than one dose of epinephrine might be needed.

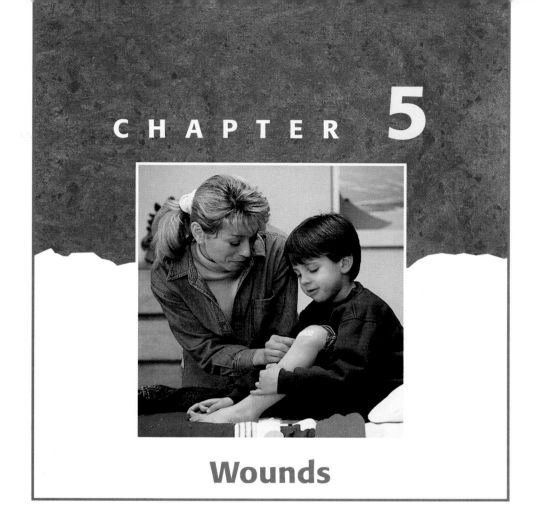

CHAPTER 5

Wounds

When an injury to the skin occurs, the first and natural concern is to stop or control the bleeding. Once that is accomplished, what remains is a fresh wound that, if properly cared for, will heal in a timely manner with a minimal risk of infection. Sometimes a wound can appear to be more serious than it actually is because of the amount of blood that you see. This is why stopping the bleeding is the first important step of wound care because, after bleeding is controlled, you can see the wound and more accurately determine how large or deep it is.

Dressings and Bandages

For many children, a colorful adhesive bandage (such as a Band–Aid™) can go a long way toward easing the upset that a minor skin wound can cause. A larger wound, however, might need a *dressing* and a *bandage*. These two terms are often used interchangeably. Although they work together, they are two separate components of the coverings applied to an open wound. The size and location of a wound determines the types of dressing and bandage necessary.

A *dressing* is a sterile pad, which is placed directly over a wound, covering it completely. It is best to stock commercial dressings, such as regular gauze pads, nonstick gauze pads, and adhesive bandages because they come in a variety of sizes, are lint-free, and are packaged sterile. The purpose of a dressing is to control bleeding and absorb drainage. It also helps to keep the wound clean and protects it from further injury.

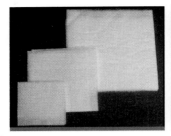

Gauze pads used for wound dressings

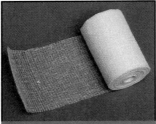

Rolled gauze bandages used to hold dressings in place

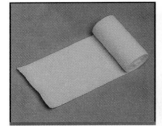

Elastic bandages used to apply compression to an extremity

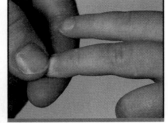

Capillary refill: check the circulation of the injured limb by squeezing the nailbed on the limb.

A *bandage* covers the dressing and holds it in place. It can also be used to apply direct pressure over a bleeding wound. A roll of wrapped gauze makes a good bandage because it can be used on any part of the body.

Elastic bandages provide compression and support to a joint or muscle and can greatly reduce swelling after an injury. Leave the tips of fingers and toes exposed so that you can check to see if the bandage is wrapped too tightly. Check for changes in color, temperature, and capillary refill in the fingers or toes of the injured limb. They should have normal skin color and feel warm to the touch. Use the capillary refill test to check circulation: firmly squeeze the child's nailbed in the injured limb. The nailbed should turn white and immediately return to the normal pink color.

DO NOT

- remove a dressing until bleeding stops. If it becomes soaked with blood, add another dressing.
- pull off a dressing that is stuck to a wound. Soak the dressing in warm tap water until it loosens.
- use cotton or a cloth with loose fibers as a dressing material, because the fibers can become caught in the wound.

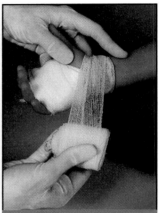
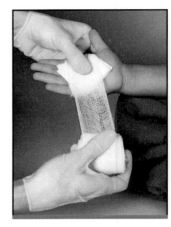
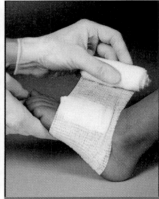
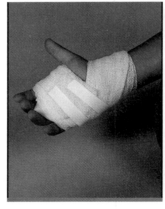
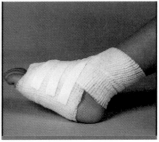
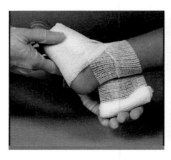

A figure-of-eight bandage secures a dressing in place on a hand or foot.

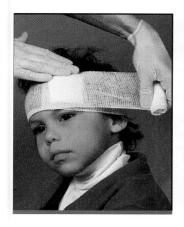
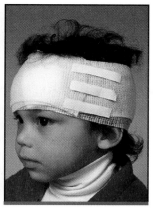

Dressing and bandaging a head wound using rolled gauze

Abrasions

An abrasion is a scrape, such as a skinned elbow or knee, that is accompanied by a small amount of bleeding or clear oozing. An abrasion is a shallow minor wound, but it can be painful if it covers a large area or is located near a joint where it is aggravated by movement.

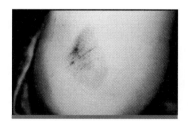

Abrasion

What to Do

1. Wear disposable gloves and wash the wound and surrounding area with soap and rinse with running water. Take care to remove all dirt and debris. Dirt left in an abrasion can leave a discolored area or stain known as a "tattoo mark" on the skin.

2. An antibacterial spray, cream, or ointment can be applied, but this is not necessary. Know your center's policy about the use of these products.

3. Leave a small, clean abrasion uncovered whenever possible.

4. Cover an abrasion that continues to bleed or needs protection because of its size or location. Use a nonstick pad or a gauze pad covered with a thin layer of petroleum jelly or antibacterial ointment to prevent the pad from sticking to

the wound. Dressings should not be airtight because they can trap moisture, which encourages bacterial growth.

5. Change the dressing if it becomes wet or dirty. Wetness draws dirt and bacteria to the wound. Remove it entirely after 24 hours, unless the wound is likely to be bumped or stressed.

6. If the dressing becomes stuck to the wound, remove it by soaking it in warm water to soften the scab. Pulling a scab loose while changing a dressing can be painful; it also slows healing and increases the chance of infection.

Lacerations

A laceration is a deep cut that bleeds freely and can have jagged and irregular edges. Deep lacerations can damage the underlying muscles, nerves, and tendons.

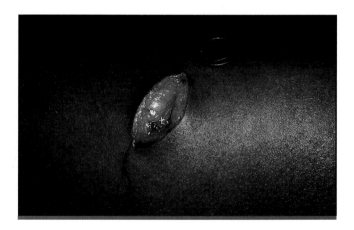

Laceration

What to Do

1. Wear disposable gloves and remove any clothing covering the wound.

2. Use direct pressure, elevation, and pressure points, as needed, to control bleeding.

3. Clean a superficial laceration with soap and water. Take care to remove all dirt and debris. Rinse the wound well and dry it.

4. Check the need for suturing, or stitches. To do this, gently try to separate the edges of the laceration. If the edges can be easily separated, if the laceration is deep or jagged, or if it is located on the face, it might need to be closed with stitches. It is not always easy to tell if a

wound needs stitches. See *About Stitches,* and call the child's parent if you are concerned.

5. Leave a small clean wound uncovered whenever possible.

6. Apply a nonstick pad, or a gauze pad covered with a thin layer of petroleum jelly or antibiotic ointment to prevent the pad from sticking to the wound. A dressing should not be airtight because it can trap moisture, which encourages bacterial growth.

DO NOT

*   attempt to clean a deep or large laceration that has clearly separated edges. These lacerations need suturing and will be thoroughly cleaned by a health care provider. Cover the laceration with a dressing and contact the child's parent.
*   use merbromin (Mercurochrome™), thimersol (Merthiolate™), iodine, or isopropyl alcohol. These products can sting and irritate the skin, and some can cause allergic reactions.

About Stitches

A large deep wound or one that continues to bleed needs to be stitched, or sutured, to reduce the risk of infection, promote healing, and decrease scarring. The size of the wound as well as the location on the body help to determine if stitches are necessary. This should be decided by a health care provider within 4 to 6 hours after the injury. If more time passes, the edges of the wound begin to heal separately, making rejoining them difficult. Without sutures, the wound will heal more slowly, increasing the likelihood of infection and scarring.

Puncture Wounds

A puncture wound is an injury from a sharp object that pierces the skin and penetrates the tissue underneath. The entrance wound is usually small. Puncture wounds can easily become infected, because they generally do not bleed and do not benefit from the cleansing effect that bleeding provides. Also, puncture wounds are sometimes so deep that air does not reach them, and bacteria can become trapped inside. Many strains of bacteria, including tetanus, thrive under such conditions.

Tetanus

Tetanus is a grave disease that causes strong, painful spasms in the back, arms, legs, and jaw—hence its other name, "lockjaw." The disease is usually fatal. Fortunately, however, because of widespread immunization, most residents of the United States are immune to the disease; in this country, there are only about 100 deaths from tetanus each year, far below the world average.

Tetanus bacteria live in soil, dust, and human and animal feces. They are usually introduced into the human body by a sharp object that pierces the skin, but they can enter through any opening in the skin that becomes contaminated with material containing the bacteria. Puncture wounds, because they can be deep and are difficult to clean, are the most likely wounds to become infected with tetanus bacteria. Furthermore, puncture wounds close, and tetanus bacteria are trapped inside where they thrive in an environment with little or no oxygen. In this environment, tetanus bacteria produce a toxin that attacks the central nervous system and brain.

Tetanus can be completely prevented through immunization. Immunization enables the immune system to manufacture its own antitoxin against a future exposure to tetanus. Children should receive a series of five tetanus immunization injections by the age of 6. They should receive a booster in the early adolescent years, and then every 10 years thereafter. Immunizations are the best defense against tetanus.

Puncture wounds can vary from minor wounds caused by a splinter, staple, safety pin, or thumbtack to more severe wounds from sharp scissors, fishing hooks, or knives.

What to Do

1. Use tweezers to remove objects that are barely penetrating or loosely hanging.

2. Clean minor puncture wounds with soap and water. Encourage a small amount of bleeding by gently squeezing the area while washing.

3. Call the child's parent if the wound is deep and the child needs to be seen by a health care provider. The child's health care provider will want to examine and clean the wound and ad-

minister a tetanus booster if the child has not had one within the last 5 years.

4. Secure in place a deeply embedded object, such as a pair of scissors, with a large, bulky, dressing. Place the child on the left side in the recovery position and treat for shock. Call for emergency medical help, as needed.

DO NOT

- remove an object that is deeply embedded because this can cause further bleeding.

Watching for Signs of Infection

In the course of healing, many small wounds develop superficial infections that the body's defenses can handle alone. Occasionally, however, even a wound that receives the most careful treatment develops a serious infection requiring medical treatment.

Try to keep all dressings clean and dry and observe a wound daily for signs of a developing infection. Call the child's parent if you observe any of the following signs and symptoms of infection.

- Throbbing pain
- Swelling
- Pus formation
- Skin around the wound that is warm to the touch
- Redness around the wound
- Red streaks leading away from the wound
- Enlarged lymph nodes
- Fever

Avulsion and Amputation

An avulsion is a partial tearing of body tissue. An amputation is the complete severing of a body part. Both injuries damage the skin, muscles, tendons, nerves, bones, and blood vessels. It is sometimes possible for an avulsed or amputated body part to be surgically repaired, if it receives proper first aid care and is reattached within a few hours after the injury. Examples of injuries that can result in avulsion or amputation are an animal bite that tears a child's nose or cheek and a finger slammed in a heavy door.

What to Do

1. Wear disposable gloves and use direct pressure, elevation, and pressure points, as needed, to control bleeding.
2. Treat for shock, if necessary. With the child on the back, raise the legs 8 to 12 inches, but no more, and cover the child with a blanket or a jacket to prevent heat loss.
3. Monitor the ABCDs and treat accordingly.
4. Rinse an amputated part, but do not scrub or clean it.
5. Wrap an amputated part in dry gauze, or another available dry, clean cloth, and place it on but not in a bed of ice.
6. Have the child seen immediately in an emergency medical facility.

DO NOT

- clean or scrub an amputated body part, because cleaning and excessive handling might damage the torn tissue.
- bury an amputated body part in ice.

Bleeding under a Fingernail

A child who catches a finger in a closing drawer or door or who receives a direct blow to the tip of a finger might have bleeding under the fingernail. This causes pressure and can be quite painful. It is easily relieved by making a hole in the surface of the nail, but this should be done by a health care provider.

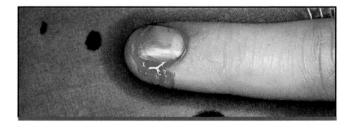

Finger slammed by door

Nail Avulsion

A nail avulsion is when a fingernail or toenail becomes partially torn away from the nailbed. Apply an adhesive bandage coated with an antibi-

WOUNDS

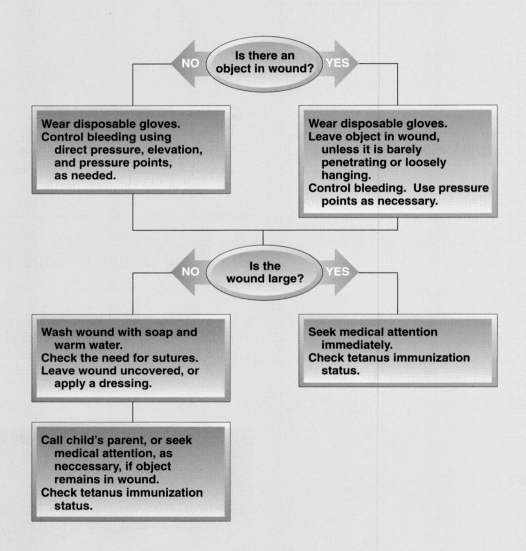

Is there an object in wound?

NO →

Wear disposable gloves.
Control bleeding using
 direct pressure, elevation,
 and pressure points,
 as needed.

YES →

Wear disposable gloves.
Leave object in wound,
 unless it is barely
 penetrating or loosely
 hanging.
Control bleeding. Use pressure
 points as necessary.

Is the wound large?

NO →

Wash wound with soap and
 warm water.
Check the need for sutures.
Leave wound uncovered, or
 apply a dressing.

Call child's parent, or seek
 medical attention, as
 neccessary, if object
 remains in wound.
Check tetanus immunization
 status.

YES →

Seek medical attention
 immediately.
Check tetanus immunization
 status.

otic ointment, and secure the damaged nail in place. Change the bandage if it becomes wet or dirty. A new nail will begin to grow in to replace the damaged nail in about 1 month. It takes approximately 4 months for a fingernail to completely grow in and 6 months for the nail on the great toe. The parent should trim the damaged nail if necessary. If the child is uncomfortable because blood has accumulated under the nailbed, the parent should call the child's health care provider.

Splinters

Most splinters are minor nuisances. If a splinter is protruding above the skin surface, remove it by grasping one end with a pair of clean tweezers and pulling it out. Do not dig with a needle to remove a splinter, because it will cause discomfort and might be unsuccessful. A deeper splinter will work itself out in several days. To reduce injuries from splinters, check all wooden playground equipment and climbing structures several times a year for areas that are splintering and have them sanded promptly.

Name _____ Course _____ Date _____

1. Circle true (T) or false (F) for each statement about wounds.

    T   F   a. If a dressing becomes stuck to a wound, you can remove it by soaking it in warm water.

    T   F   b. Apply an airtight bandage over a minor wound to prevent infection.

    T   F   c. A wound can be sutured up to 24 hours after the injury.

    T   F   d. Dressings and bandages should be changed if they become wet or dirty.

    T   F   e. Wounds are sutured primarily to reduce infection and scarring.

    T   F   f. Clotting begins after the heavy flow of blood is reduced.

    T   F   g. One dose of tetanus vaccine provides immunization for a lifetime.

    T   F   h. Immediately washing a wound with soap and water helps to prevent infection.

Check the best answer for the following questions regarding types of wounds:

2. A skinned elbow or knee is an example of which type of wound?

    ____ a. Incisions

    ____ b. Avulsions

    ____ c. Lacerations

    ____ d. Abrasions

3. Which type of wound has a jagged, irregular edge?

    ____ a. Incisions

    ____ b. Lacerations

    ____ c. Bruises

    ____ d. Puncture wounds

4. Which type of wound is caused by a sharp, pointed object, such as a thumb tack or splinter?

    ____ a. Abrasions

    ____ b. Avulsions

    ____ c. Punctures

    ____ d. Lacerations

5. Which type of wound is most likely to need sutures?

    ____ a. A puncture wound from a human bite

    ____ b. A puncture wound from a thumb tack

    ____ c. A laceration from a sharp can

    ____ d. An abrasion from a fall off a bicycle

6. Circle yes (Y) or no (N) for the following statements.

    Placing a dressing over a cleaned laceration will:

    Y   N   a. Eliminate the need for stitches.

    Y   N   b. Keep the wound clean and dry.

    Y   N   c. Prevent shock.

CHAPTER 6

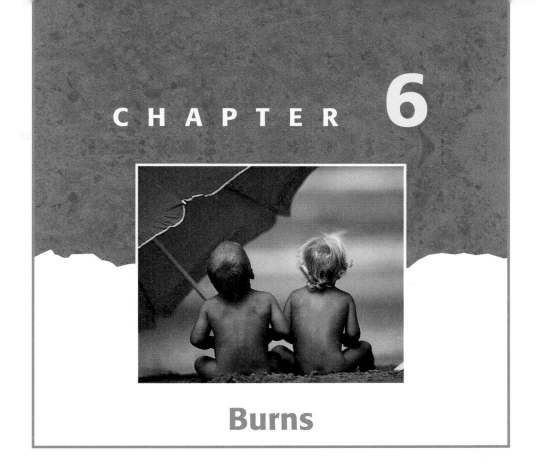

Burns

A serious burn injury can leave a child with long-term physical and emotional scars. Curious children climb and grab; they do not have a clear understanding of what is dangerous; and they are fascinated by fire. The National Institute of Burn Medicine estimates that between 50% and 90% of all burns that occur in children under the age of 4 years could be prevented! Most burns to toddlers and preschoolers are scald injuries caused by hot liquids and grease. Flame burns more commonly occur to children aged 5 to 12 years.

Many burn injuries can be prevented if you make burn-proofing a part of child-proofing in your home or center. Do you always place hot coffee out of a child's reach? Are your matches always returned to a safe, high, and hidden location? Are you teaching the children in your care that fire is a tool, not a toy?

The skin is sensitive to heat. Temperatures below 111°F generally do not damage the skin. Temperatures above 111°F cause significant tissue damage, and temperatures above 123°F destroy skin within seconds. Some states have a policy on water temperature limits in a child care setting. Know your state's policy.

Did You Know?

More than 27,000 children are hospitalized each year with burn injuries. An estimated 400,000 more are treated in emergency rooms, physicians' offices, and clinics. More than half of all childhood burns occur to children under the age of 4 years.

Source: National Institute of Burn Medicine, Ann Arbor, Michigan.

Preventing Burn Injuries

In the Bathroom

- Set the temperature of the hot water heater at 120°F. Test the water temperature with a candy or meat thermometer.

- When filling the tub for an infant or young child, run the hot and cold water together at the desired temperature. Then turn off the hot water first, so the faucet becomes cool. Test the temperature again before putting the child into the water. Do not put the child in until all water is turned off.

- Supervise toddlers and young children in the bathtub. If left unattended, they could scald themselves by turning on the hot water.

- Mark the hot water faucet with red fingernail polish or paint, and teach children that this means "don't touch." Also, use a plastic sponge cover on the tub faucet to prevent children from touching the faucet when hot.

In the Bedroom

- Keep cribs a safe distance from radiators and electrical outlets.

- Do not use extension cords in a child's bedroom. Position lamps and other items that use electricity in front of the wall outlet. This helps to eliminate the child's interest in both electrical cords and outlets.

- Cover unused outlets with plastic covers.

- Do not use a space heater in a child's bedroom.

Electrical Appliances

- Use only electrical appliances approved by Underwriters Laboratory (UL).

- Keep all electrical kitchen appliances at the back of the kitchen counter and unplugged when not in use.

- Keep electrical appliances away from water.

- Do not allow electrical cords to snake along a countertop or dangle over the edge. Loosely coil electrical appliance cords, so that children cannot pull on them. Regularly check for frayed or damaged electrical cords.

- Cover electrical outlets with plastic covers to prevent children from sticking metal items, such as pins or narrow keys, into them.

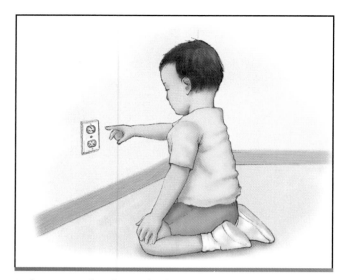

Make sure outlets have plastic covers.

- It is best not to use extension cords around infants and toddlers. If you must, keep them out of sight. A child can be electrocuted by biting through a live electric cord. If used, do not overload extension cords.

- Do not run extension cords under rugs in areas of heavy traffic.

- Never leave a hot iron unattended. Unplug and remove it before you walk away.

In the Kitchen

- Cook on back burners whenever possible to prevent children from touching a hot electric coil or lighted gas burner. When cooking on front burners, turn pan handles inward to prevent them from being knocked over or pulled down.

- Remove stove knobs when they are not in use.

- Teach children the meaning of "hot."

- Test foods and formula warmed in a microwave oven. Foods can be warmed unevenly, creating hot spots.

- Supervise children when they are ready to learn to cook.

- Do not store foods that children like to get for themselves, such as cereal, over a stove.

- Do not place any hot liquids near the edge of a table or counter.

- Use place mats set back from the edge of the table rather than tablecloths that can be pulled, causing hot liquids and dangerous items to fall.

- At meals, never pass a hot liquid or dish over a young child's head.

Outdoor Cooking

- Use only charcoal lighter fluid to light charcoal. Never use gasoline or any other flammable liquid.
- Never squirt charcoal lighter fluid on a burning fire, because it might ignite the entire can of fluid, causing the can to explode and resulting in burns.
- Keep the grill away from flammable walls and fences.
- Teach children to stay away from a grill that is in use.
- Do not throw hot embers on the ground or sand, because a barefooted child might step on them.

Fire Prevention

- Teach your children that fire burns.
- Be firm about keeping matches or lighters out of the reach of young children. Parents should teach older children how to use matches and lighters safely.
- Do not overload the electrical circuits with multiple extension cords.
- Install smoke detectors and keep them operating properly. Check the batteries in the spring and fall when you change your clocks.
- Install smoke detectors on each floor of your home or center. At least one detector should be located within 6 feet of each bedroom. Some experts now recommend that a separate detector also be placed in every bedroom in which people sleep with the door closed. Critical minutes can be lost while the smoke from one room reaches the detector in a hallway. Place a kitchen smoke detector a few feet away from the kitchen, because even a small amount of smoke from the toaster can trigger the alarm. In the construction of new buildings, smoke alarms are interconnected and powered by electricity so that if one alarm detects smoke, they all react.
- Have a fire escape plan for your family, with a designated place to meet outside the house. Have a realistic plan for how everyone can get out of his or her bedroom window. Install fire escape ladders, if necessary. Hold a practice fire drill.
- Discard flammable liquids and oily cloths properly and promptly after use. Never store them near a heat source.
- If you smell gas or suspect a gas leak, open a window or door for fresh air and immediately leave the building. From another building, call the fire department first and then the gas company. Do not turn an electric switch on *or* off and do not light a match.
- Place barriers around wood stoves, and place screens in front of fireplaces.
- Make certain that everyone knows the location of the fire extinguisher. Do not store it where

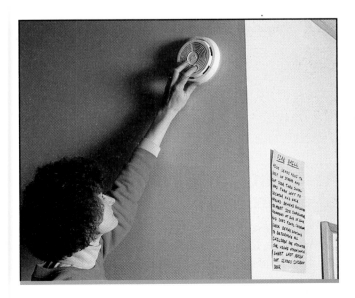

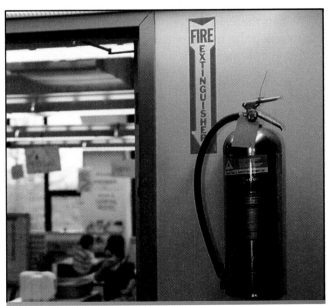

Cris, age 6, was helping his mother decorate the Christmas tree when he accidentally leaned back into a table decoration, with candles, and ignited his sweatshirt. Cris had watched the Firebusters program and remembered to "Stop, Drop, and Roll" when your clothes catch fire. He was not injured as a result of his actions.

Five-year-old Abby, asleep in the mobile home of the grandparents she and her cousin were visiting, awoke at 1:00 a.m. to find fire and smoke in her room. Frightened as she was, Abby remembered the Learn Not to Burn presentation at her school a few months earlier. Abby dropped to the floor and crawled the length of the 65-foot home to awaken her grandparents and cousin. All four escaped unharmed, although the home was completely destroyed.

Kate, age 8, responded successfully to an early morning fire in her home. The fire had cracked windows with its heat, setting off the burglar alarm. Hearing this, Kate woke up coughing to a home filled with smoke. Her bedroom door was closed. Kate reacted quickly. Crawling on her hands and knees, she moved over to the door and felt the knob. It was hot. Kate then crawled back to her sleeping sister and woke her up. After breaking the window with a rocking chair, as her father had taught her in their home escape planning, Kate made sure her sister was safely outside before leaving the burning house herself.

Marcus, age 9, was in the bathtub when he heard his six-year-old brother yelling. Jumping from the tub, he discovered that the younger brother had set his clothing on fire while playing with a lighter. Marcus first threw his towel at him. Realizing that this was not extinguishing the flames, he ordered his brother to "Stop, Drop, and Roll." The local fire department had presented two fire safety programs at Marcus's school in the previous six months.

Celelana's family's three-story apartment house was the target of an incendiary fire. When a smoke detector alerted her mother to the danger, she instructed her daughter to get out quickly. Six-year-old Celelana located her four-year-old sister, crying in her bedroom from fear of the smoke, and pulled her to the floor. She told the younger girl, "We must crawl under smoke to get out." Their mother found them both sitting on the grass in the front of the house, which was by then engulfed in flames. Celelana told her she had learned the steps she followed from "Fireman Friendly" at her school.

Source: **National Fire Protection Association, Quincy, Mass.**

---

you would most likely need to use it: beside the oven, fireplace, or wood stove. You might not be able to get to it when you need it.

- When they are old enough, teach children how to reach the fire department in your community by telephone.

What Causes Burns

Heat burns are the most common burn injury in young children. They are caused by contact with flames and other hot sources such as hot liquids and grease and appliances.

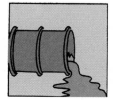

Chemical burns are caused by corrosive chemicals, many of which are stored in garages and basements.

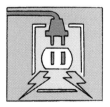

Electrical burns are caused by contact with household current or with lightning, which can cause other injuries as well.

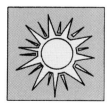

Ultraviolet rays from the sun burn unprotected skin.

Assessing the Severity of a Burn

The severity of a burn is determined by three major factors: size, location, and depth. The age of the child and pre-existing medical conditions also influence the seriousness of the injury and the recovery.

Children should know where the fire extinguishers are located. Extinguishers should be used only by a trained adult and only if the fire is small and contained.

Children should know the fire escape plan of their child care center. It should be posted in every room and practiced. There should be two ways of exiting each room and a place where everyone meets outside. Do not go back inside for any reason.

Children should know to use stairways, not elevators, when leaving a burning building.

Children should know to tie long hair back and not to wear loose-fitting clothes while cooking or standing next to an open flame. Hair and clothing can easily catch on fire.

Children should know that neither they nor their friends should play with matches or lighters. Instruct children to tell a teacher or parent if they find any.

Children should know the phrase, "Stop, drop, and roll." This will remind them to smother flames on their clothing by dropping to the ground and rolling. Running when clothes catch on fire helps the fire burn and increases the chance of inhaling smoke and flames. Also, teach children to cover their faces with both hands when rolling.

Children should know that a fire needs air to burn. Grease fires in a kitchen should be smothered with a lid, not doused with water.

Children should know to crawl to avoid breathing smoke and poisonous fumes when leaving a burning building. The cleanest air is found low to the ground.

Children should know that if they are in a burning building and come to a closed door, they should feel it with their hands. If the door is hot, there is smoke or fire on the opposite side. Do not open it.

Children should know that if they cannot escape a burning building, they should crawl to a room that has a telephone or a window to the outside. Call the emergency rescue number in your area. Signal for help from the window if there is no fire below that window.

Children should know that they should never go into a closet or under a bed. Rescuers won't be able to find them.

Children should know that the fire safety information they know might save a life.

Children should share what they know with their friends and parents.

Size

The larger the burn area, the more serious the injury. Descriptions such as "the size of a quarter," "one side of the leg," or "half of the back" help to define the size. In children, estimating the size of a burn as a percentage is done by using the child's palm as 1% of the surface area and totalling the palm-sized areas of injured skin.

Location

Burns can be especially serious when they are located on one of the four critical areas of the body—the face, the hands, the genitals, and the feet. Unfortunately, children commonly burn these areas when they reach up to stove tops, touch hot appliances, or spill hot liquids in their laps. Flame

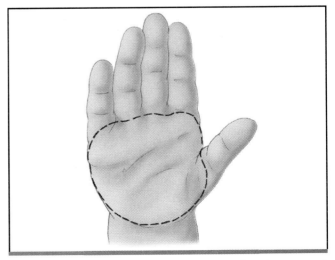

The palm of the hand equals 1% of the total surface area of the body.

burns can be especially damaging, because, in addition to the destruction of the skin, the fumes can damage the lining of the airway, causing swelling and narrowing of the breathing passages.

Age

A burn is more worrisome in an infant or a young child than in an older child or adult because the imbalance of body fluids caused by a serious burn injury is more difficult to correct in the younger child.

Pre-Existing Medical Condition

Diseases, such as heart or kidney disease, diabetes, asthma, or an immune system disorder, make it difficult for the child with a serious burn injury to recover easily and fight off infection.

Depth

Burns are currently described as superficial, partial-thickness, or full-thickness, replacing the terms first degree, second degree, and third degree. These newer terms are more descriptive of the varying depths of damage in a burn injury. The depth of a burn is deter-

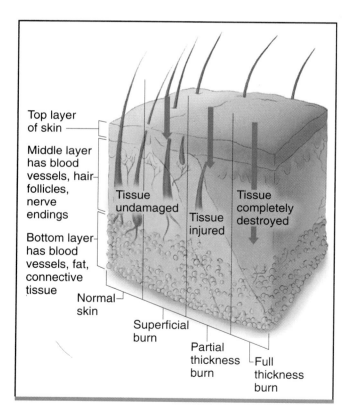

Depth of burn injury

Source: Adapted with permission from the National Institute for Burn Medicine, Ann Arbor, MI.

mined by the temperature as well as the length of time that the burning substance is in contact with the skin.

What to Look For

Superficial Burn
This burn causes minor skin damage.

- Skin pink or red
- Mild swelling, no blisters
- Pain, but it is mild in comparison to partial-thickness burn pain
- Heals completely within a few days

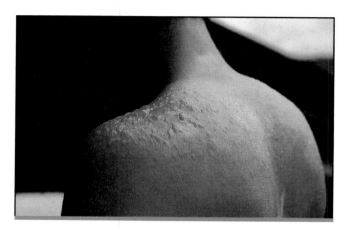

Partial-thickness burn: blistered shoulders

Partial-Thickness Burn
This burn damages, but does not completely destroy, the full depth of skin.

- Dark red or bright red
- Blisters
- Swelling
- Severe pain
- Might take a few weeks to heal

Full-Thickness Burn
This burn severely damages or destroys the full depth of skin, hair follicles, muscle, nerves, and other tissue.

- Red, raw, ash white, black, leathery, or charred
- Swelling
- Little or no pain in area of full-thickness damage because nerves are destroyed. Pain results from surrounding partial thickness and superficial burn areas.
- Almost always requires skin grafting, because the skin cannot regenerate after a burn of this depth. Skin grafting is a surgical procedure that

transplants healthy skin from another part of the body to the area where skin is destroyed.

What to Do

For most burn injuries, immediate first aid action can limit the extent of the damage. Delayed or improper first aid allows a burn injury to become more severe, increases the risk of infection, and slows healing.

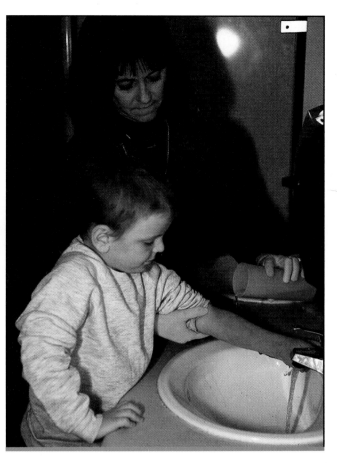

Cooling the burn with water

First Aid for All Burns

- Stop the burning process.
- Cool the burn with water, regardless of the source of the burn.

1. Stop the burning process.
   - Heat burns—Remove the child from the source of heat. If flames are present, smother them by using a blanket or rolling the child on the floor or grass. Prevent the child from running because this fans the flames and helps the fire burn.
   - Chemical burns—Brush off any dry chemical that remains on the skin.
   - Electrical burns—Be sure the child is no longer connected to the source of the electricity. Turn off the power source before approaching the child.
   - Ultraviolet radiation burns—Bring the child indoors.
2. Cool the burn with water.
   - Wear disposable gloves and place all burn-injured skin in cool water, or cover with a cold, wet towel if you cannot get the burn area into a container of water, such as with a burn on the face. Avoid using forceful running water. If using a towel, saturate it every 1 to 2 minutes to keep it cold. This treatment cools the tissues and helps to dull the pain for the first few hours after a burn.
   - If the burn is caused by a chemical, use running water for 10 to 15 minutes to rinse the area. Avoid using a forceful flow, because this can drive the chemical into the skin.

3. Remove surrounding clothing while saturating the burned area. Some synthetic materials melt onto the skin and are difficult to remove. If clothing adheres to the skin, do not try to remove it.
4. Contact the child's parent or call for emergency medical help, depending on the extent of the burn injury. Call your local poison control center for advice about a chemical burn injury. See *When to Seek Medical Treatment for a Burn Injury* if you are unsure.

DO NOT

- place ice on a burn, because ice damages the fragile skin that remains.
- apply ointments (including burn ointments), petroleum jelly, butter, margarine, toothpaste, or creams. These products trap the heat, causing further pain and damage.
- break blisters, because they protect the burn and prevent infection.

Flame-Retardant Fabric

The most severe burns involve burning clothing. The type of fabric a child is wearing significantly contributes to the severity of a burn. New synthetic fibers are less flammable than the more natural fibers of cotton, nylon, and wool but create more damaging burns because the material actually melts onto the skin. In 1972, a federal law was passed requiring all children's sleepwear, sizes infant through 6X, to be flame-retardant. This law has substantially reduced the burns caused by flames in younger children. The flame-retardant chemicals that are applied to clothing, however, can be removed if not laundered properly.

To protect the flame-retardant quality of children's clothing:

- Wash in warm water with a phosphate detergent only, not a laundry soap.
- Never use bleach or fabric softeners.
- Drip dry or tumble-dry on low settings.
- Do not iron.

When to Seek Medical Treatment for a Burn Injury

If you are unsure of the severity of the burn and whether medical treatment is necessary, consult the following list of guidelines. The child should be seen immediately by a health care provider if:

- Burn pain is severe enough that the child is inconsolable and unable to be distracted.
- The child is under 5 years of age with a partial-thickness burn larger than the size of a quarter.
- The child has a full-thickness burn of any size.
- The child has a pre-existing medical condition.
- There are partial-thickness or full-thickness burns on the child's face, hands, feet, or genitals or the burn encircles an arm, leg, or the chest.
- The burn was caused by a chemical.
- Another injury accompanies the burn.
- The child might have inhaled smoke or flames.
- Signs of abuse are present, such as cigarette burns, a clear border of submersion on a burned extremity, or a burn injury with an explanation that does not seem plausible.

Unprotected in the Sun—Is It Worth the Risk?

Unprotected skin is exposed to the harmful ultraviolet rays of the sun whether the day is sunny or cloudy. Repeated exposure to the sun causes early aging of the skin and changes that can allow skin cancers to occur later in life. Skin can be damaged by ultraviolet rays whether burning or tanning, and the harm from repeated unprotected and underprotected exposures is cumulative.

A mild sunburn is usually a superficial burn and is characterized by redness, pain, and tenderness, especially when trying to move the burned area. It can worsen as the day progresses, even hours after coming inside. A more serious sunburn is a partial-thickness burn and is characterized by blisters on the burned area, chills, nausea, and pain that can be so intense that the child will not tolerate clothing on the area.

Relieving the Pain of Sunburn

To help relieve the discomfort of a child's sunburn, use cool water liberally. Apply over-the-counter sunburn remedies to nonblistered skin, if desired.

These products do not speed healing, but they soothe the skin. Give a mild analgesic, such as acetaminophen, to help relieve pain. Consult the child's health care provider concerning a sunburn that blisters or if the child has any of the symptoms that accompany a more severe sunburn.

Sunburn Precautions

We now know that the summer sun is not as friendly as the warm rays make us feel it is. Protecting skin from the sun is essential to avoid sunburn now and to protect against the long-term damage that years of exposure to ultraviolet rays can produce.

- Limit children's exposure to direct sunlight between the hours of 11:00 AM and 3:00 PM, when the sun's rays are the most intense.
- All children should wear a sunscreen with a sun protection factor (SPF) of at least 15, regardless of the skin's tanning ability. The SPF number indicates the amount of protection the product

BURN INJURIES

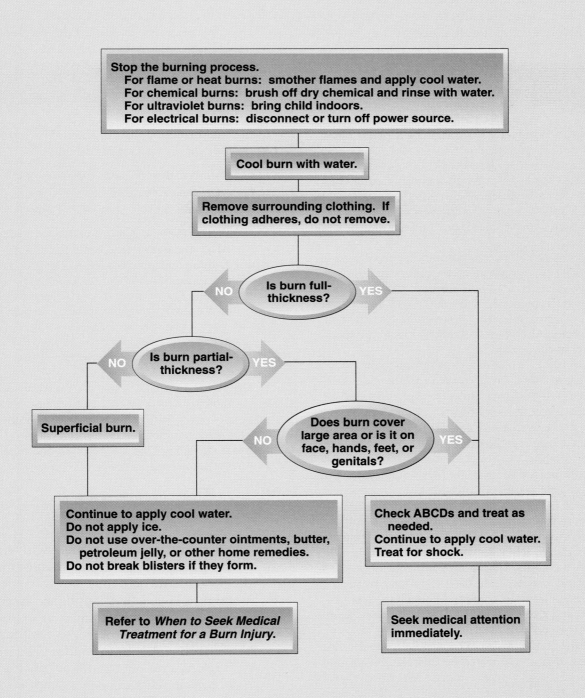

Stop the burning process.
    For flame or heat burns: smother flames and apply cool water.
    For chemical burns: brush off dry chemical and rinse with water.
    For ultraviolet burns: bring child indoors.
    For electrical burns: disconnect or turn off power source.

Cool burn with water.

Remove surrounding clothing. If clothing adheres, do not remove.

Is burn full-thickness?
NO   YES

Is burn partial-thickness?
NO   YES

Superficial burn.

Does burn cover large area or is it on face, hands, feet, or genitals?
NO   YES

Continue to apply cool water.
Do not apply ice.
Do not use over-the-counter ointments, butter, petroleum jelly, or other home remedies.
Do not break blisters if they form.

Check ABCDs and treat as needed.
Continue to apply cool water.
Treat for shock.

Refer to *When to Seek Medical Treatment for a Burn Injury.*

Seek medical attention immediately.

provides. The higher the number, the greater the protection.

- Choose sunscreens that block both UVA and UVB rays, because they provide protection against the widest range of ultraviolet rays.
- Apply sunscreen liberally to frequently exposed areas, such as the face, the back of the neck, the shoulders, behind the knees, and the tops of the feet. There are sunscreen products made exclusively for children that do not sting sensitive skin. Do not apply any sunscreen products to a rash or an open cut.
- Apply sunscreen 20 to 30 minutes before going outside. This allows the protective ingredients time to be absorbed below the surface of the skin. Reapply sunscreen often when out-of-doors. Even products that claim to be waterproof can be washed away by playing in water or sweating.
- The reflection of ultraviolet rays off the water at a pool, lake, or ocean and off the sand at the

Exposure to Indoor Electricity

When used properly, electricity is one of our safest and cleanest sources of power. Because its use is so routine, we tend to forget the enormous energy potential behind the seemingly innocent household outlet. Even a household current of 110 volts can be deadly under certain conditions, such as using an appliance with wet hands or while standing on a wet floor.

Electricity follows the path of least resistance. In the body, this path is along the nerves and through the body fluids. Electrical current enters a child's body at the point of contact and travels rapidly, generating heat and causing destruction. Usually the electricity exits where the child is touching a metal object or the ground.

Electrical current that passes through the body can cause severe damage or life-threatening injuries, such as full-thickness burns or respiratory and cardiac arrest. It can also ignite clothing. Even though the burn injury appears to be small, the internal damage can be extensive. Recovery can take many months.

Most indoor electrical injuries result from the use of faulty electrical appliances or from improper or careless use of electrical equipment. Electrical injuries to young children are typically the result of biting through an electrical cord or sticking a metal paper clip or safety pin into a wall outlet.

Most children who receive an electrical shock are knocked away from the electrical source by the force generated from the contact. Although the child is upset and shaken, there are no lasting effects from this type of shock.

If the child remains in contact with the electrical source, it is a life-threatening emergency. The child is termed "hot" with electricity: the electricity will be transmitted to anyone who touches the child. Electricity causes strong muscle contractions that result in the child holding on tightly to the damaged elec-

trical cord or faulty appliance. The child is unable to let go until the electricity is turned off.

Electricity travels best in water—the body of a child is more than 75% water.

National Institute for Burn Medicine, Ann Arbor, Michigan

Should this ever happen to a child in your care, go directly to the power source and turn off the power. Unplug the appliance if the plug is undamaged and you can reach it without coming in contact with the child. Otherwise, turn off the electricity by using the wall switch, circuit breaker, fuse box, or outside switch box. Everyone should know where the main power source is located and how to turn it off. Approach the child *only* after the power source has been disconnected.

Any child who sustains a severe electrical shock needs immediate medical attention because of the possibility of respiratory or cardiac arrest. In this event, the burn injury, even if full-thickness, becomes secondary. Check the ABCDs and treat accordingly. Send someone to call for emergency medical help.

NEVER

- touch a child who is in contact with electricity via a faulty cord or appliance until the power is turned off.
- attempt to kick a "hot" appliance away from a child who is holding it or to push it away with another object, even if the object is thought not to conduct electricity, such as a broom handle, because it is risky to yourself and your attempt is likely to be ineffective.

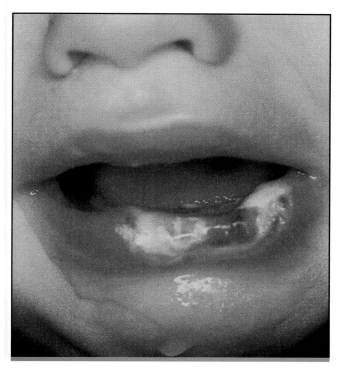

Full-thickness electrical burn injury from biting through an electrical cord

- Children under the age of 1 year require special protection. They should have almost no exposure to direct sun and should not be taken to a beach. If exposed to direct sun, they should have all skin covered with clothing and wear a hat. Manufacturers of sunscreens recommend that their products not be used on infants under the age of 6 months.

- Some antibiotics can increase a child's sensitivity to the sun's rays. Check medication containers for warning labels.

- Do not tell a child that a tan is a sign of good health or beauty. It is important to educate even young children about the risks of sun exposure to prevent unnecessary sunburns now and sun-related health problems later in life.

beach increases the intensity of the sun's rays. When in these locations, use cover-ups, such as shirts, hats, and an umbrella.

Downed High-Voltage Electrical Lines

Although electrical wires are infrequently downed, adults should know how to proceed safely when dealing with this very dangerous situation. *Never* attempt to move downed wires unless you are trained and equipped with tools capable of safely handling high voltage.

If a child is trapped in a car with an electrical line fallen across it, tell the child to stay in the car and keep hands folded in the lap. To prevent electrocution, the power must be disconnected by the electric company before the child can be allowed to get out of the car. Stand at least 15 feet from the car and prevent bystanders from entering the dangerous area immediately surrounding the vehicle.

This is an example of a situation in which it is unsafe for a first aider to approach an injured child. Outside help is necessary from the electric company before first aid can be started.

Avoiding Lightning

The most important defense against being injured by lightning is to know when and where lightning is likely to occur and be alert during those times and in those places. Lightning occurs most often between May and September, and almost 75% of lightning injuries and deaths occur in the afternoon. Protect the children in your care and your family by being respectful of the power of lightning, and avoid getting in its path.

If you are indoors when a storm approaches, you should stay there. Do not take a bath or a shower or use the telephone, because they can conduct electricity.

If you are caught outdoors when a storm approaches, you should take shelter in a sturdy building. If none is available take cover in a hard-top automobile and close the windows. If you are not near any shelter, take cover under a group of small trees, but stay away from a tall or isolated tree, because it can act like a lightning rod and stands a greater chance of being hit by lightning. Stay away from bicycles, golf carts, motorcycles, and farm equipment.

If you are in or on any body of water, such as a swimming pool, ocean, lake, river, or stream, you should get out and away at the first rumble of thunder. A good rule of thumb is if you can hear thunder, you are close enough to the storm to be struck by lightning. Do not return to the water until 20 minutes after the last rumble of thunder.

Name _____ Course _____ Date _____

1. Circle true (T) or false (F) for each of the following statements about burns.

   T   F   a. Temperatures below 111°F generally do not damage the skin.

   T   F   b. Some states have a policy on water temperature limits in a child care setting.

   T   F   c. Ultraviolet rays from the sun do not burn skin.

   T   F   d. First aid for all burns includes cooling the burn with water.

   T   F   e. To reduce pain and promote healing, both petroleum jelly and burn ointment are beneficial.

   T   F   f. Full-thickness burns almost always require skin grafting.

   T   F   g. For many burn injuries, applying ice can limit the extent of the damage.

   T   F   h. A child should be seen by a health care provider for a full-thickness burn of any size.

2. The severity of a burn is determined by three major factors. These are:

   a. _____

   b. _____

   c. _____

3. Two-year-old Jonathan reaches across the table when your attention is elsewhere and pulls a cup of steaming hot coffee across the table and into his lap. Circle yes (Y) or no (N) for each statement about caring for a burn.

   Y   N   a. Remove his clothing if it comes off easily.

   Y   N   b. Apply cold water to cool the skin.

   Y   N   c. Break any blisters that form to relieve pressure.

   Y   N   d. Apply a burn ointment, petroleum jelly, or butter to soothe the burned skin.

4. Circle true (T) or false (F) for each of the following statements.

   T   F   a. Some antibiotics can increase a child's sensitivity to the sun's rays.

   T   F   b. The sun's rays are the strongest between the hours of 2:00 PM and 5:00 PM.

   T   F   c. Only children with light skin need to wear sunblock.

   T   F   d. The reflection of the sun on water or sand increases the intensity of the rays.

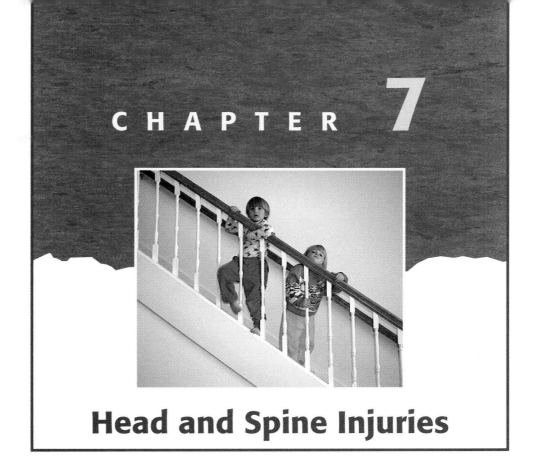

CHAPTER 7

Head and Spine Injuries

Injuries to the head and spine can be the most devastating injuries that the body can sustain, because these injuries can affect the ability to make decisions, communicate ideas, and to control body movement. With the passage of time, wounds, burns, and broken bones will heal. But the same cannot always be said of head and spine injuries. Some injuries to the brain and major nerves of the spine result in damage so severe that function cannot be restored to the preinjury state no matter how much time and medical care is devoted to recovery.

Head Injuries

Head injuries are common during the childhood years. Most are superficial, with bruising and swelling of the skin, such as a "goose egg," but some can be severe enough to cause permanent brain damage or death. The Centers for Disease Control estimates that falls account for more than half of all head injuries to children under the age of 5. After the age of 5, head injuries are caused equally by sports, falls, and motor vehicle accidents.

Did You Know?

- *Almost 30% of all childhood injury deaths result from head injuries.*
- *Each year, an estimated 29,000 children suffer permanent disability from moderate or severe head injury.*

Statistics taken from the Centers for Disease Control: Childhood Injures in the United States, *June 1990.*

Bump on the Head

During the first few years of life when young children are learning to crawl, climb, and walk, small bumps on the head are an everyday occurrence. Because there is little soft tissue surrounding the skull to absorb the blood and other fluids from such injuries, blood collects under the skin in one bulging area often referred to as a "goose egg." A child with a minor bump on the head does not lose consciousness. Apply ice or a cold pack wrapped in a wet cloth to control swelling and, just to be safe, observe for signs and symptoms of internal head injury. See *Internal Head Injury* in this chapter.

Scalp Wound

The seriousness of a wound on the head can be deceiving, because the head has such a rich supply of blood vessels that even minor wounds tend to bleed heavily. However, because of this blood supply, cuts on the head rarely become infected.

What to Do

1. Raise the child's head and shoulders.
2. Control bleeding. Wear disposable gloves and apply gentle direct pressure to the wound. Bleeding should stop in 5 to 10 minutes.
3. Apply ice or a cold pack wrapped in a wet cloth to control swelling.
4. Clean a minor scalp wound with soap and water and determine the need for stitches. See *About Stitches* in Chapter 5.
5. Observe for signs and symptoms of internal head injury.

Internal Head Injury

Internal head injury refers to damage inside the skull. When the head receives a forceful blow, the brain smashes against the skull, resulting in some degree of injury, which can range from minor bruising to permanent brain injury. The accumulation of blood and other fluids inside the skull exerts pressure against the brain, because the bones of the skull cannot expand to make room for the bleeding and swelling that accompanies this type of injury.

Concussion is a term that generally refers to the symptoms of dizziness, nausea, and a loss of consciousness after a violent jarring of the brain. Unconsciousness can last for just a few seconds or for as long as several days.

Cold Pack Alternatives

Some ways to apply cold to an injured area to reduce swelling after an injury include:

1. Crushed ice in a baggie.
2. Wet washcloth placed in a baggie and kept in the refrigerator.
3. Commercial "snap pack" ice packs.
4. Frozen vegetables and other frozen foods.
5. Popsicle placed directly on the skin when treating an injury inside the mouth.

Never place cold packs directly against a child's skin. Always wrap the cold pack in a cloth to protect the skin.

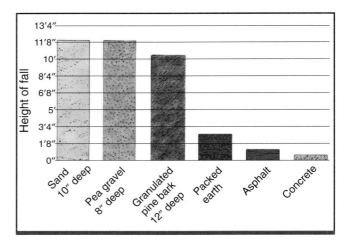

This graph shows the approximate height from which a falling child would sustain internal head injury on each playground surface.

Source: Franklin Research Center, Norristown, Pa.

Since internal head injury can be present even in the absence of a visible skull wound, the following signs and symptoms are the most reliable indicators of internal head injury.

What to Look For

- Unconsciousness. A child might appear stunned for several seconds after a head injury, but this is not the same as unconsciousness.
- Confusion or memory loss. A child can be upset after a head injury but should know where he or she is and what happened.

- Agitation or combativeness
- Nausea and vomiting
- Severe headache lasting several hours
- Blurred vision
- Dizziness or difficulty with balance
- Pale, sweaty appearance
- Unusual sleepiness
- Pupils of unequal size. The small, black, round centers of the child's eyes should be of equal size and should become smaller when exposed to light.

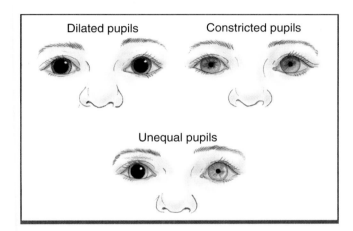

- Clear fluid (cerebrospinal fluid) or blood dripping from the nose or collecting in the ear(s)
- Seizure
- Swelling of an infant's soft spot—the fontanel— located on the top of the head
- Skull depression. A depressed skull fracture is most often seen in infants.

What to Do

1. Check for responsiveness by calling the child's name. Check and monitor the ABCDs and treat accordingly. A child who loses consciousness after a violent head injury should be treated as if he or she has a spine injury. See *Spine Injuries* in this chapter.
2. If the child is responsive, raise the head and shoulders. This decreases pressure on the brain.
3. If a wound is present, apply gentle direct pressure to control bleeding. See *Scalp Wound* in this chapter.
4. Apply ice or a cold pack wrapped in a wet cloth to control swelling.
5. Observe the child for signs and symptoms of an internal head injury for 24 to 48 hours.

6. Contact the child's parent immediately if the child shows any signs or symptoms of internal head injury or a depressed skull fracture. Even a child who only loses consciousness for 5 to 10 seconds should be examined in an emergency medical facility.

DO NOT

- **give anything to eat or drink until the child is well enough to continue a normal routine.**
- **give any pain medication, including acetaminophen, aspirin, or ibuprofen, to a child with a head injury unless instructed to do so by a health care provider.**

A child who does not lose consciousness after hitting the head and who quickly returns to normal activity is probably fine. If you are uncertain of the child's condition, contact the parent and have the child seen by a health care provider.

Sleeping after a Head Injury

A child who has had a head injury may be allowed to sleep if it is the normal naptime or bedtime. However, do not allow a child to sleep for longer than 2 hours without being awakened. The child should be easily arousable. Sleeping does not worsen the child's condition. The concern is that a sleeping child cannot be observed for changes in behavior and level of consciousness.

Special Considerations about Infants and Head Injuries

An infant's skull has fontanels, also called "soft spots," where the bones have not yet grown together. Infants are especially vulnerable to head injuries, because the skull bones are fragile and the brain is not protected in the area of the fontanels. Therefore, a blow to the head of an infant should always be examined by a health care provider even if, initially, there are no signs of internal injury.

Eye Injuries
Chemical Injury to the Eye

Chemicals get into children's eyes most commonly from products in spray bottles, such as household cleaners and pesticides. A chemical burn to the eye requires immediate first aid treatment to prevent

HEAD INJURIES

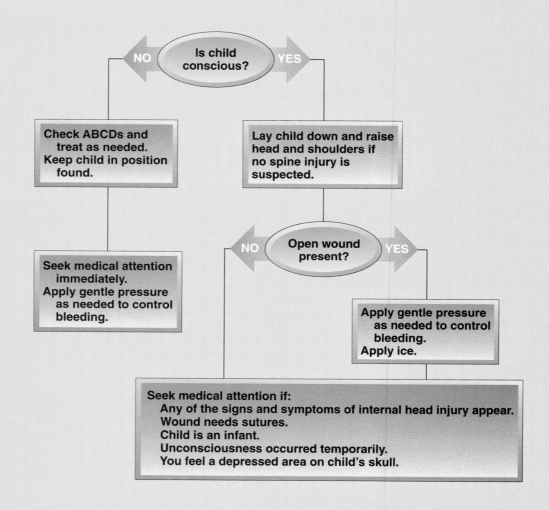

Is child conscious?

NO

Check ABCDs and treat as needed. Keep child in position found.

Seek medical attention immediately. Apply gentle pressure as needed to control bleeding.

YES

Lay child down and raise head and shoulders if no spine injury is suspected.

Open wound present?

NO

YES

Apply gentle pressure as needed to control bleeding. Apply ice.

Seek medical attention if:
   Any of the signs and symptoms of internal head injury appear.
   Wound needs sutures.
   Child is an infant.
   Unconsciousness occurred temporarily.
   You feel a depressed area on child's skull.

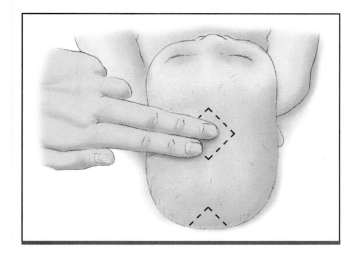

Location of infant fontanels (soft spots)

damage to the cornea, the transparent outer covering of the eyeball. Eye damage can occur swiftly—in less than 5 minutes. An eye that appears only slightly red initially can quickly develop deeper damage, depending on the chemical and the length of exposure.

What to Do

1. Wear disposable gloves and immediately flush the chemical from the eye with warm water. Position the head over a sink with the injured eye down to prevent the rinse water from contaminating the other eye. Hold the injured eye open with your fingers and pour water into the eye from an unbreakable cup for 15 minutes. Rinse from the inside of the eye toward the outside. You may need to securely wrap a young child in a large towel to help hold the child still.

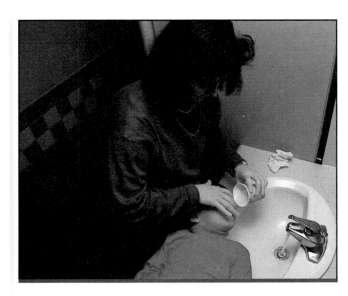

Flush a chemical from an eye with warm water.

2. Call the poison control center to find out what further care the eye needs.
3. Loosely dress and bandage both eyes if the child needs to be seen by a health care provider.

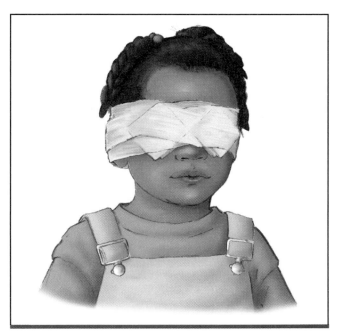

Bandaging both eyes

This will protect the injured eye from unnecessary movement, because both eyes move in unison.

4. Notify the child's parent.

Penetrating Injury to the Eye

Most penetrating eye injuries are obvious. However, you should also suspect penetration whenever an eye lid is cut. A penetrating injury requires immediate ophthalmologic attention.

What to Do

1. Wear disposable gloves and cover the injured eye and the object with a paper cup to prevent further penetration. Rest the cup on several thick gauze pads and tape it in place. Also place a gauze pad over the uninjured eye. This will protect the injured eye from unnecessary movement, because both eyes move in unison. Wrap a rolled gauze around the head several times securing the coverings over the eyes.
2. Keep the child flat on the back.
3. Have the child seen in an emergency medical facility immediately.
4. Call the child's parent.

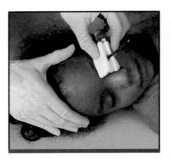
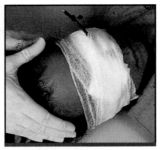

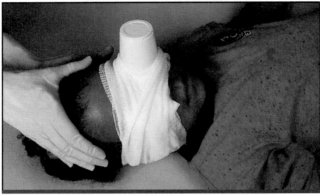

Securing in place an object penetrating the eye

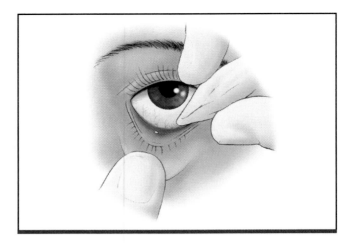

Remove a small floating object with the corner of a clean, white cotton handkerchief.

DO NOT

- attempt to remove a foreign object penetrating the eye.

Foreign Object in Eye

Eye lashes, dirt, insects, and bits of sand are foreign objects that commonly cause discomfort and tearing of the eyes. Discourage a child from rubbing the eyes, because this can scratch the cornea, the transparent outer covering of the eyeball. A corneal scratch is painful, damages the cornea, and can introduce infection.

What to Do

1. Wear disposable gloves. Pull down the child's lower eyelid and look at the inner surface while the child looks up. A speck of dirt or a insect can usually be removed with the corner of a clean, white cotton handkerchief. If you cannot see the object, it might be under the upper lid.

2. Gently grasp the upper lid and pull it out and down over the lower eyelid. This is often helpful in dislodging the object.

3. If the object remains, flush the eye with warm water. Position the head over a sink, injured eye down. Hold the eye open with your fingers and

pour water into the eye from an unbreakable cup. Rinse from the inside of the eye toward the outside.

4. Call the child's parent. The child should be examined by a health care provider if the eye continues to be red, tearing, or painful. The foreign body might have scratched the cornea, the surface of the eye, and this injury can only be confirmed with a special dye and lamp. A child with a scratched cornea might need an antibiotic ointment and an eye patch.

DO NOT

- allow the child to rub the eye, because this could scratch the cornea.
- use cotton swabs or tissues, because they can deposit fibers in the eye.

Cut on the Eye or Lid

Keep the child in a semi-sitting position. Wear disposable gloves. Cover both eyes with a gauze pad and bandage loosely. Do not attempt to flush the eye with water or apply pressure to the injured eyelid. Call the child's parent to have the child seen in an emergency medical facility.

Blow to the Eye

Gently place ice or a cold pack wrapped in a wet cloth around the injured eye for 10 to 15 minutes to control swelling and reduce pain. A black eye or blurred vision might indicate internal eye damage, and the child should be seen by an ophthalmologist as soon as possible.

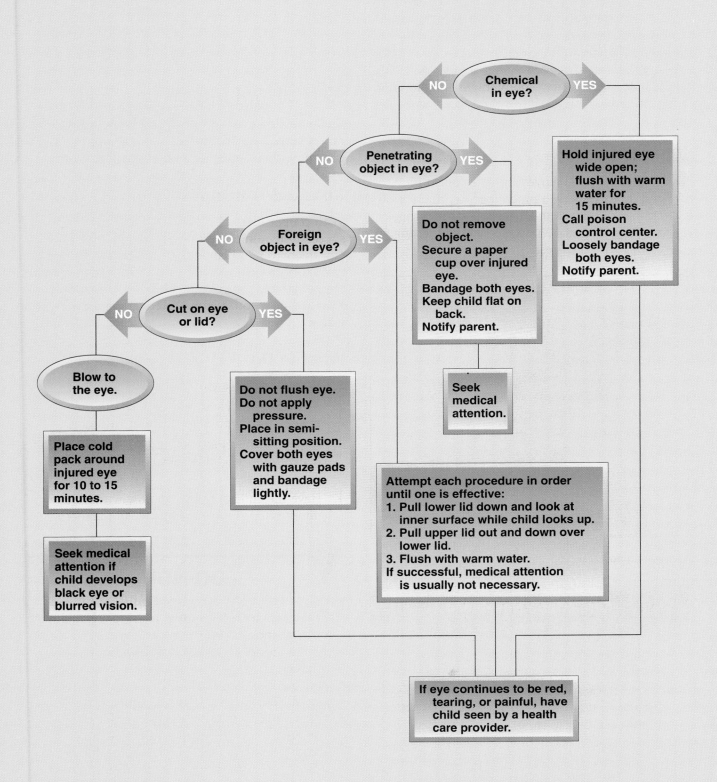

Chemical in eye?
- NO
- YES → Hold injured eye wide open; flush with warm water for 15 minutes. Call poison control center. Loosely bandage both eyes. Notify parent.

Penetrating object in eye?
- NO
- YES → Do not remove object. Secure a paper cup over injured eye. Bandage both eyes. Keep child flat on back. Notify parent. → Seek medical attention.

Foreign object in eye?
- NO
- YES → Attempt each procedure in order until one is effective:
  1. Pull lower lid down and look at inner surface while child looks up.
  2. Pull upper lid out and down over lower lid.
  3. Flush with warm water.
  If successful, medical attention is usually not necessary.

Cut on eye or lid?
- NO
- YES → Do not flush eye. Do not apply pressure. Place in semi-sitting position. Cover both eyes with gauze pads and bandage lightly.

Blow to the eye.
- Place cold pack around injured eye for 10 to 15 minutes.
- Seek medical attention if child develops black eye or blurred vision.

If eye continues to be red, tearing, or painful, have child seen by a health care provider.

Nosebleed

Nosebleeds are generally more annoying than serious, especially in a young child. It is the abrupt appearance of a nosebleed that alarms adults. A bump to the nose, crying, laughing, and picking at the nose can all cause a nosebleed. Spontaneous nosebleeds are more common during the colder months, when both indoor and outdoor air is dry. Bleeding can seem heavier than it actually is; a tissue that appears very bloody might contain only a tiny amount of blood. If the child received a direct, forceful blow to the nose, suspect a fracture.

What to Do

1. Wear disposable gloves and use your thumb and index fingers to pinch together the nostrils on the soft part of the nose below the bridge. Squeeze for 5 to 10 minutes, without letting go to check the progress.

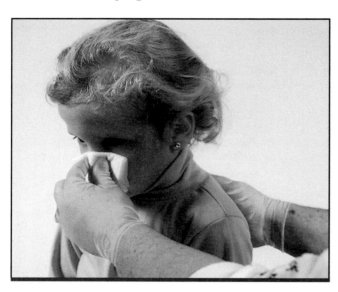

Caring for a nosebleed

Care after a Nosebleed

- Encourage the child not to pick or rub the nose.
- Keep the nostrils moist by using saline nose drops or applying a little petroleum jelly just inside the nostrils twice a day.
- Use a cool mist vaporizer in the child's sleeping area when air is dry during the winter months.

2. Tilt the head forward so that the blood runs out of the nose rather than down the throat. Blood is irritating to the stomach and can cause nausea and vomiting.
3. Call the child's parent if the bleeding cannot be controlled after 30 to 45 minutes. Parents should discuss frequent, unprovoked nosebleeds with the child's health care provider.

Dental and Mouth Injuries

The following first aid procedures provide temporary relief for dental injuries, but it is important to consult with a dentist as soon as possible.

Knocked-Out Tooth

With proper first aid a knocked-out tooth can be successfully reimplanted in the socket. It is important to try to reimplant a baby tooth as well as a permanent tooth, because it acts as a space saver for the permanent tooth. A knocked-out or partially knocked-out tooth is considered a dental emergency.

What to Do

1. Wear disposable gloves.
2. A partially knocked-out tooth should be pushed back into place without rinsing it.
3. A knocked-out tooth should be placed in a container with the child's saliva or whole milk to keep it moist.
4. Have the child seen by a dentist within 30 minutes to improve the chance of the tooth surviving.

DO NOT

- **use lowfat milk, powdered milk, or milk products, such as yogurt, to keep a knocked-out tooth moist.**
- **put the tooth in mouthwash, water, or alcohol.**
- **scrub a knocked-out tooth.**
- **touch the root of a knocked-out tooth.**
- **ask a child to place the tooth under the tongue to keep it moist while waiting to see the dentist. This method is acceptable for adults but risky for young children, because the tooth can be swallowed accidentally.**

NOSEBLEED

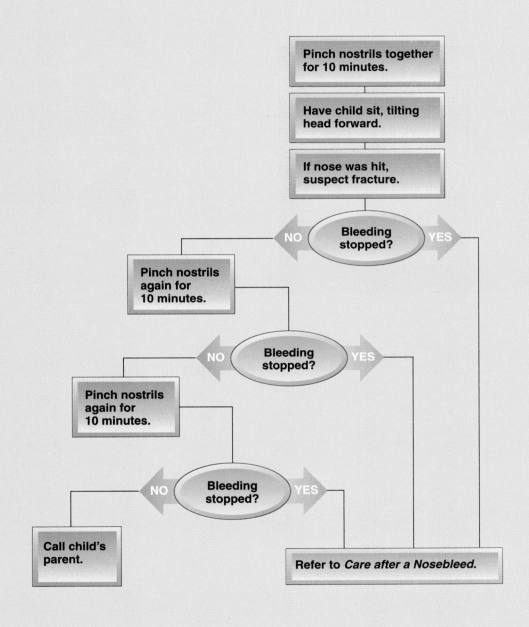

Pinch nostrils together for 10 minutes.

Have child sit, tilting head forward.

If nose was hit, suspect fracture.

Bleeding stopped?

NO → Pinch nostrils again for 10 minutes.

YES → Refer to *Care after a Nosebleed.*

Bleeding stopped?

NO → Pinch nostrils again for 10 minutes.

YES → Refer to *Care after a Nosebleed.*

Bleeding stopped?

NO → Call child's parent.

YES → Refer to *Care after a Nosebleed.*

Broken Tooth

A child who breaks a tooth should be seen by a dentist immediately, because the break can extend down to the root of the tooth. For a simple chipped tooth, a dentist will file off sharp edges to prevent the child from cutting the lip or tongue. If the injury extends to the root, the tooth might need more extensive dental work. Have the child rinse with warm water to clean the tooth and apply ice or a cold pack wrapped in a wet cloth against the face to decrease swelling.

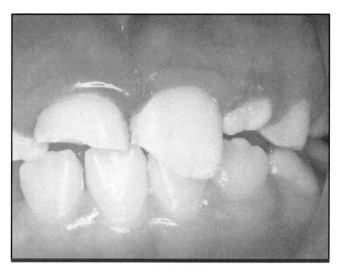

Broken teeth

Bite to the Tongue or Lip

Although it is a common injury to young children, damage from a bite to the tongue or lip can be difficult to assess. The mouth has a rich supply of blood vessels and cuts tend to bleed heavily. The amount of bleeding is deceiving, because when blood mixes with saliva, there appears to be more blood than there actually is. Stitches are seldom used when treating cuts of the mouth, unless the wound is large, because the mucous membrane of the tongue and of the inside of the mouth is delicate and tears easily.

What to Do

1. Have the child rinse the mouth with water.
2. Keep the child in a sitting position.
3. Wear disposable gloves and apply pressure with a piece of gauze or a clean cloth to stop the bleeding.
4. Apply ice or a cold pack wrapped in a wet cloth to control the swelling.

5. Call the child's parent and recommend that the child be seen by the health care provider if the cut is deep and extends from the lip to the skin surrounding the lip or if there is a gaping cut on the tongue with persistent bleeding. This cut will probably need stitches.

Toothache

If a child complains of a toothache, put on disposable gloves and rinse the child's mouth with warm water. Use dental floss to remove any food that might be caught. A cotton ball saturated with oil of clove placed on the tooth can relieve some discomfort. If pain continues, call the child's parent to recommend that the child be seen by a dentist.

Object Wedged between Teeth

Occasionally children complain of food caught between the teeth. Most often these particles can be removed by gripping the object with a piece of clean gauze or a dry tissue. If this is unsuccessful, use a piece of dental floss to remove the object from between the child's teeth. Do not use a sharp pointed object, such as a toothpick, to remove debris. Always wear disposable gloves when touching the inside of a child's mouth.

Foreign Objects

It should be common practice to keep small objects out of the reach of young children, because of the risk of choking. Be aware that some children put tiny objects, such as beads, buttons, bits of food, plant parts, and pencil-top erasers, in their noses and ears.

In Ears

You should suspect a foreign body in a child's ear canal if the child pays unusual attention to the ear but does not appear to be in pain. The child might also confide that there is something in the ear. Do not try to remove the object with cotton swabs or tweezers because a young child cannot be relied upon to hold still and the skin of the ear canal is delicate and can be easily damaged . A health care provider can easily remove the object with special tweezers or a warm water ear flush.

DENTAL INJURIES

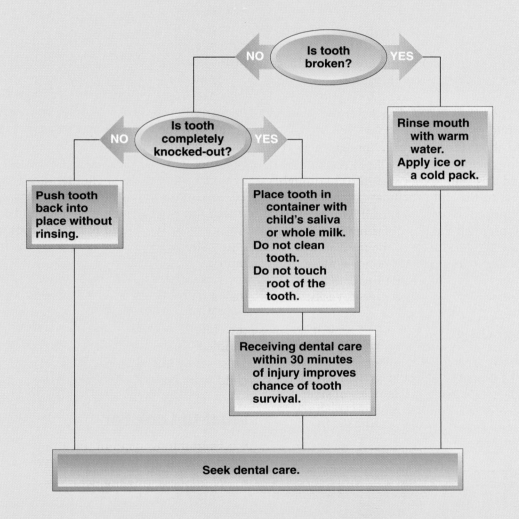

Is tooth broken?

NO

YES

Rinse mouth with warm water.
Apply ice or a cold pack.

Is tooth completely knocked-out?

NO

YES

Push tooth back into place without rinsing.

Place tooth in container with child's saliva or whole milk.
Do not clean tooth.
Do not touch root of the tooth.

Receiving dental care within 30 minutes of injury improves chance of tooth survival.

Seek dental care.

If a child becomes aware that a live insect is in the ear canal, either because the child feels it or hears a buzzing sound, assure the child that the insect cannot travel any farther inside the body. A teaspoon of lukewarm vegetable oil poured into the ear canal kills the insect, but this procedure should not be attempted if the child has surgically implanted tubes in the ears. If this treatment is unsuccessful, contact the child's parent and recommend that the child been seen by a health care provider. Never try to remove an insect by inserting a cotton swab or any other object into the ear canal.

In Nose

A foreign object in the nose develops a foul odor and causes a one-sided runny nose within a few hours. The child might pick at the nose if the object is annoying or if it interferes with nasal breathing. It is not unusual for a child to have a foreign object caught in the nose for several days before telling a parent or a child care provider.

The child should try to expel a foreign object by gently blowing the nose but only if old enough to have mastered this skill. Otherwise, the child might sniff the object further into the nose. Do not attempt to remove the object yourself with tweezers because this can push the object farther into the nose. The moist environment of the nose allows some objects to expand, making removal more difficult. All clinics and health care providers have special tweezers to remove these objects easily.

Swallowed Objects

Except for sharp items, small objects swallowed by a child pass through the digestive system without complications in 3 to 4 days. Examples of such normally harmless objects are buttons and small toy pieces. A parent might want to call the health care

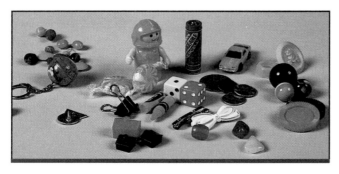

Children sometimes swallow tiny objects or put them in their noses or ears.

provider if there is any question about the danger of a swallowed object. The local poison control center is also a good source of information. Watch for the swallowed object to appear in the child's stool. Do not give a laxative. Although unusual, if abdominal pain develops during the following few days, the parent should call the child's health care provider.

Spine Injuries

A spine injury damages the bony spinal column that surrounds and protects the nerves of the spine, known as the spinal cord. These nerves allow us to feel sensations and to move our bodies. Any serious injury to the spinal column and nerves can cause paralysis, or permanent loss of feeling and movement, below the area of the injury.

Spine fractures are becoming increasingly common in children. They most often result from the bending, twisting, or jolting movements that occur with the violent impact of a motor vehicle or bicycle accident or from a sports-related injury. In fact, motor vehicle accidents are the leading cause of spinal cord injury in children under the age of 16, followed by sports-related injuries, acts of violence (almost all from gunshot wounds), and falls. Any child who is found to be unresponsive after an injury should be treated as if he or she has a spine injury.

It is important to be aware that the nerves inside the spinal column might remain undamaged even if a bone in the spine is fractured. However, if the child is allowed to sit up or is improperly handled, the spinal nerves can become damaged. This is why immobilizing the neck and spine of a child with a suspected spine injury is so important.

What to Look For

- Painful movement of the arms and/or legs. Pain can be sharp or radiate down the arm or leg.
- Numbness, tingling, weakness, or a burning sensation in the arms or legs
- Paralysis of the arms or legs
- Deformity, or unnatural position, of the child's head and neck

What to Do

1. If the child is unresponsive, first check for breathing in the position in which the child is found. Try to determine if the child is breathing

by putting your face close to the child's face and listening and feeling for breaths. If the child is not breathing or if you cannot tell, then you must roll the child onto the back as one unit. Open the airway by lifting the chin only. This is unlikely to aggravate a neck or spine injury. Continue to check the ABCDs and treat accordingly.

2. If the child is responsive, tell the child not to move. Immobilize the head, neck, and spine by padding with towels, blankets, or jackets.

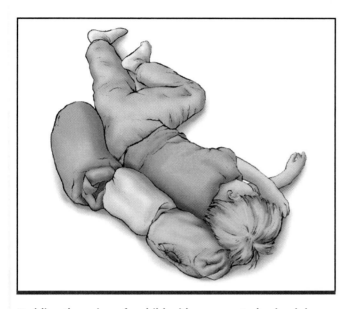

Padding the spine of a child with a suspected spine injury

3. If the child begins to vomit, roll as one unit on to the left side into the recovery position.

4. Send someone to call for emergency medical help.

5. If the injury occurs in a swimming pool or other body of water, strap the child to a back board before removing from the water.

DO NOT

- move or change the position of a child with a suspected spine fracture, unless an emergency forces you to do so.

6. Arrange for transportation to an emergency medical facility immediately.

SPINE INJURIES

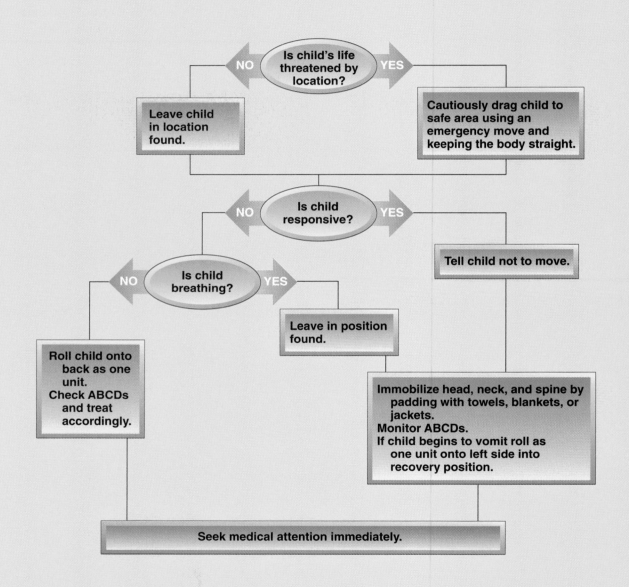

Is child's life threatened by location?

NO → Leave child in location found.

YES → Cautiously drag child to safe area using an emergency move and keeping the body straight.

Is child responsive?

YES → Tell child not to move.

NO →

Is child breathing?

YES → Leave in position found.

Immobilize head, neck, and spine by padding with towels, blankets, or jackets.
Monitor ABCDs.
If child begins to vomit roll as one unit onto left side into recovery position.

NO → Roll child onto back as one unit.
Check ABCDs and treat accordingly.

Seek medical attention immediately.

STUDY QUESTIONS 7

Name _____ Course _____ Date _____

1. Circle true (T) or false (F) for the following statements about head injuries.

   T F a. Head injuries are not as worrisome in infants as they are in children, because infants have fontanels.

   T F b. Scalp wounds tend to bleed very little.

   T F c. Confusion can be a symptom of internal head injury.

   T F d. Do not allow a child to sleep for longer than 8 hours after a head injury.

   T F e. Do not give any pain medication to a child who complains of a headache after a head injury.

2. At a neighborhood playground, a child throws a rock that hits the head of another child. The injured child is crying and has a bleeding wound on his forehead. Which of the following first aid measures should you take? Circle yes (Y) or no (N) for each statement.

   Y N a. Clean the wound with soap and water.

   Y N b. Have the child lie flat.

   Y N c. Apply a warm pack to control swelling.

   Y N d. Control bleeding with direct pressure.

3. List four signs or symptoms that would lead you to believe that the child described in question 2 might have an internal head injury.

   a. _____

   b. _____

   c. _____

   d. _____

4. Circle true (T) or false (F) for each of the following statements about eye injuries.

   T F a. Rubbing the eye helps to remove a foreign object without damaging the cornea.

   T F b. If the eye appears to be all right after first aid treatment for a chemical in the eye, it is unlikely that there is damage.

   T F c. Rinse an eye by pouring warm water from the inside part of the eye toward the outside.

   T F d. Blurred vision after a blow to the eye is common and does not indicate serious injury.

5. Circle yes (Y) or no (N) for the following statements about care for nosebleeds.

   Y N a. Have the child sit and tilt the head backward.

   Y N b. Pinch the nostrils for 2 to 3 minutes.

   Y N c. Call child's parent if bleeding cannot be controlled after 30 to 45 minutes.

6. Complete the following statements by filling in the blanks.

   a. While arranging an emergency visit to the dentist, place a child's knocked-out tooth in _____ or _____.

   b. A child should be seen by a dentist within _____ of having a tooth knocked out.

   c. You would suspect that a child has a foreign object in the nose if the child_____
   _____.

   d. Except for sharp items, small swallowed objects usually pass through a child's digestive system in _____ days.

7. Circle true (T) or false (F) for the following questions about spinal injuries.

   T F a. Serious injury to the spinal cord causes paralysis.

   T F b. Do not move a child with a suspected spinal injury unless an emergency forces you to do so.

   T F c. Loss of movement in the arms and hands might indicate nerve damage in the neck or upper spine.

   T F d. A child who is found unconscious after a violent injury must be treated as if a spinal injury has occurred.

   T F e. It is possible to have a spinal fracture without damaging the spinal cord.

   T F f. Motor vehicle accidents are the leading cause of spinal cord injury in children under the age of 16.

CHAPTER 8

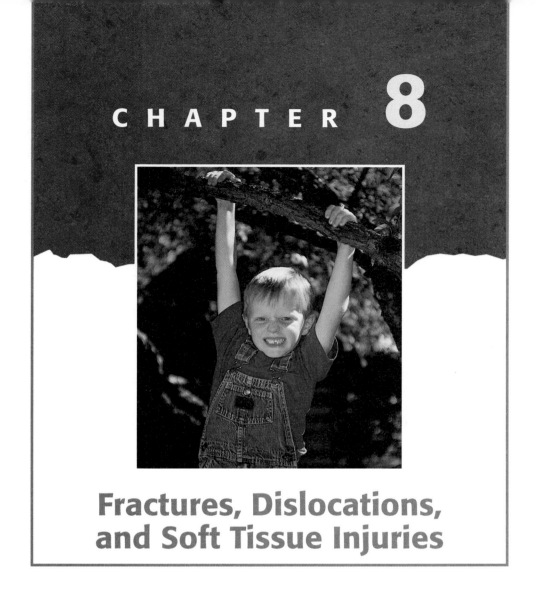

Fractures, Dislocations, and Soft Tissue Injuries

The bones and joints of young children have not yet been subjected to the normal wear and tear that comes with aging and are generally more flexible than those of adults. Because of this flexibility, children rarely strain or tear muscles as adults commonly do while stretching, bending, running, jumping, or twisting. But flexibility has its disadvantages. Young children are more prone to dislocations of the joints, especially of the elbow, than are adults. Also, because of their activity level, enthusiasm, and, at times, impulsive behavior they commonly experience broken bones and soft tissue injuries such as bruises.

Fractures

A fracture is a broken bone. A fracture can be a partial break or a complete break in the bone caused by a twist or a direct blow. Fractures are common in children. They can be of concern if there is damage to the growth plate, the area of the bone where growth takes place, because damage in this area can cause irregular growth and shortening of the bone. Fractures can also involve damage to the surrounding muscles, nerves, and blood vessels. Fortunately for children, bone healing after a fracture is more rapid than in adults. This is because their bones have a more generous blood supply and because the thick and strong outer covering of their bones contains more bone-forming cells than do adult bones.

Knowing with certainty that a bone is broken is not always possible just by looking at it. This is why an x-ray of a suspected broken bone is always taken to confirm that it is fractured and to get a more detailed look at the bone.

Types of Fractures

- *Closed (simple) fracture.* The skin is not broken where the bone is fractured.

- *Open (compound) fracture.* There is an open wound over the fracture caused by either the bone breaking through the skin or by the force of the trauma. The bone is not always visible. Open fractures are more serious than closed fractures, because there is greater blood loss and a chance of infection.

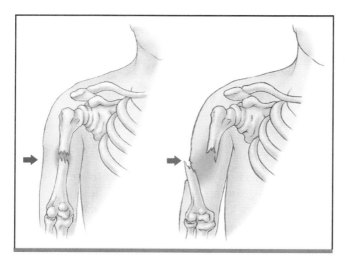

Closed fracture   Open fracture

What to Look For

- Scene suggests that traumatic injury has just occurred.

- Pain and tenderness. The child complains of a sharp pain at the site of the injury.

- Swelling. This is caused by blood and other fluids collecting around the injury.

- Deformity. Sometimes the break in the bone results in an unnatural shape or bend of the body part. Compare the injured body part with

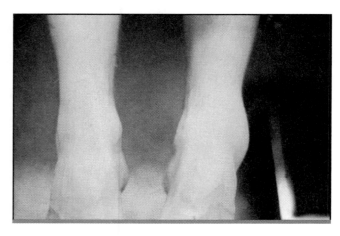

Compare injured side to uninjured side.

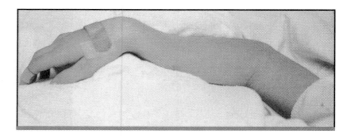

Forearm fracture

the uninjured side of the body to check for deformity.

- Loss of mobility. The child might be able to move the injured part slightly but will not have full range of motion.

What to Do

1. Remove clothing surrounding the injury to check for signs and symptoms of a fracture. Cut the clothing, if necessary to avoid moving the injury. Ask the child what happened and to point to where it hurts.

2. Look for swelling, tenderness, or deformity.

3. If a wound is present, wear disposable gloves and control bleeding, as necessary. Apply pressure at a pressure point if the bone is protruding through the skin, which prevents you from applying direct pressure. Cover the wound with a sterile dressing or large clean cloth to keep it as clean as possible. See *Pressure Points*, Chapter 4.

DO NOT

- **attempt to clean a wound if you suspect that there is a fracture.**

4. Immobilize a suspected fracture by supporting it against the body or by padding the area with towels or pillows in the position in which the child is most comfortable. This limits movement and pain. See *About Splinting in a Child Care Center.*

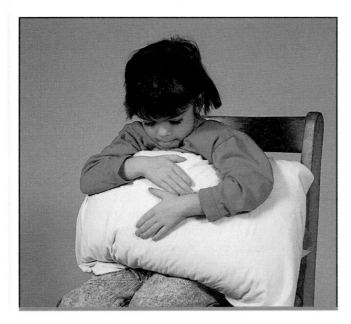

Support broken ribs with a pillow.

5. To avoid placing pressure on a fracture, place ice or cold packs wrapped in a wet cloth on both sides of an injured arm or leg rather than directly on top of it. This helps to reduce swelling and pain.

6. Elevate the injured arm or leg, if it does not cause increased pain. This also helps to reduce swelling and pain.

7. Treat the child for shock. Cover the child with a blanket to prevent heat loss.

8. Make arrangements to transport the child to a medical facility. If the injury is in a location that makes moving the child difficult, call for emergency medical help.

DO NOT

• **give anything to eat or drink.**

About Splinting in a Child Care Center

Knowing how to splint a broken bone can be useful in many situations. However, it is generally recom-

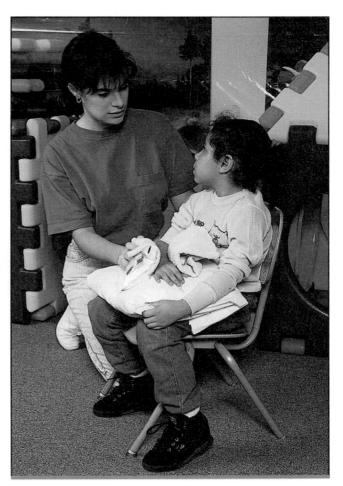

Place cold packs on both sides of the injured forearm.

mended that child care providers not splint the suspected broken bones of young children if emergency medical help is nearby, for several reasons:

- A young child in pain cannot be relied on to be cooperative.

- Splints can be applied incorrectly because of the inexperience of the first aider. A splint that is applied too tightly or positions a limb incorrectly can restrict circulation and cause further pain and damage.

- Unnecessary movement of the injury during splinting can cause additional pain and damage to the bone, soft tissue, blood vessels, and nerves.

- In a child care setting, *immobilization* of a suspected fracture by padding the injury with towels and pillows is preferred over splinting. Immobilization provides substantial stability and minimizes movement, so there is less chance of causing additional harm. It is best if emergency medical technicians apply splints to suspected broken bones. Their knowledge and expertise allows them to apply a splint easily and safely. Know your center's policy about splinting.

Dislocations

A dislocation is the separation of a bone from a joint. In children, dislocations commonly happen to fingers and elbows. It takes only a small amount of force for a child's bone to become dislocated, because children's ligaments are very flexible. A simple quick tug on a child's hand to prevent the child from stepping from a curb or to protect against a stumble can be enough to dislocate an elbow. Infants and young children should never be picked up by their hands or wrists. Always lift them by placing your hands under their armpits.

What to Look For

- Pain and tenderness. A dislocated bone can be very painful, if ligaments are torn and nerves are damaged.
- Swelling. This is caused by bleeding within the tissues.
- Deformity. This is caused by the unnatural shape of the bone outside of the joint socket. Sometimes the bone will relocate itself immediately, but often it needs to be returned to its proper position by a health care provider.
- Loss of mobility. Any movement of the joint causes pain if the bone remains dislocated.

What to Do

1. Ask the child what happened and to point to where it hurts.
2. Remove clothing surrounding the injury to check for swelling, tenderness, or a deformity. Move the injury as little as possible.

DO NOT

- **try to correct a dislocated bone yourself because blood vessels and nerves can become caught in the joint space, causing further injury.**
- **give the child anything to eat or drink.**

3. Immobilize the injury in the position in which the child is most comfortable. Allow the child to hold the injured area against the body or support the injury with a pillow or towels to prevent further movement and discomfort.
4. Apply ice or a cold pack wrapped in a wet cloth to the injured area to decrease swelling and pain.
5. Call the child's parent to have the child seen by a health care provider.

Soft Tissue Injuries

A soft tissue injury is one in which "soft" tissue structures such as ligaments, blood vessels, and muscles are damaged, resulting in pain, swelling, and decreased movement of the injured area. Examples of soft tissue injuries are sprains, muscle pulls, and bruises. In addition, some soft tissue damage always occurs when a bone is fractured or dislocated. Sometimes the soft tissue injury is so severe that the symptoms mimic those of a fractured bone.

Sprains

A sprain is a twisting of a joint, along with tearing of its supportive muscles and ligaments. Sprains are uncommon in young children because their ligaments are very flexible and stronger than their bones. Often in a traumatic injury, the bone breaks before the ligament is stressed to the point where damage occurs to it. Sprains begin to occur in children as they progress through grade school and their joints become more like adult joints.

It can be difficult to distinguish between a fracture and a sprain because the symptoms are similar. If a child in your care has an injury to a limb characterized by pain, swelling, loss of movement, and loss of use, treat the injury as if it were a fracture and arrange for the child to be seen by a health care provider.

If you do not suspect that the child has a fracture, use the following RICE procedure.

What to Do

The following first aid measures, known by the acronym RICE (which stands for rest, ice, compression, and elevation), are effective when treating soft tissue injuries, such as sprains or pulled

FRACTURES AND DISLOCATIONS

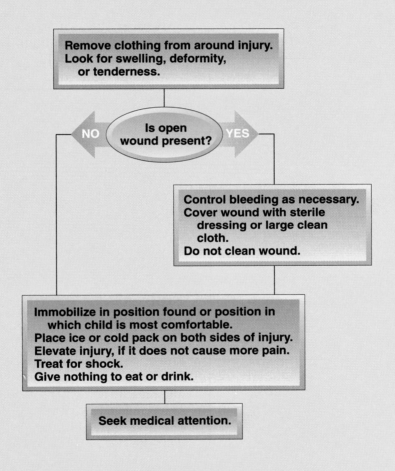

Remove clothing from around injury. Look for swelling, deformity, or tenderness.

Is open wound present?

NO

YES

Control bleeding as necessary.
Cover wound with sterile dressing or large clean cloth.
Do not clean wound.

Immobilize in position found or position in which child is most comfortable.
Place ice or cold pack on both sides of injury.
Elevate injury, if it does not cause more pain.
Treat for shock.
Give nothing to eat or drink.

Seek medical attention.

muscles, which are more commonly experienced by school-aged and older children.

1. **Rest.** Have the child sit or lie down.

2. **Ice.** Cover the injury with a wet cloth, and apply ice or a cold pack for periods of 20 minutes every 2 to 3 hours for the first 24 hours. This reduces pain, bleeding, and swelling. Placing a wet cloth directly on the skin transfers the necessary cold more effectively than a dry cloth, yet protects the skin from the extreme cold. Continuous use of ice is not recommended, because it can result in frostbite.

3. **Compression.** Compress the injured area by applying an elastic bandage. This limits the collection of blood and other fluid. Apply the elastic bandage by starting a few inches below

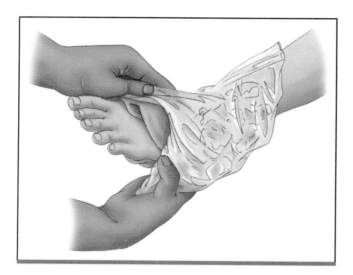

Apply ice over a wet cloth.

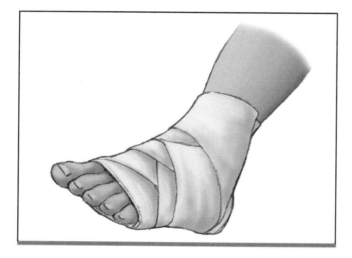

Compress the injured area by applying an elastic bandage.

the injury and wrapping upward in a spiral manner. Use firm, even pressure, making sure you do not wrap too tightly. If the child complains that the fingers or toes are cold, tingling, or becoming numb, loosen the bandage. Leave the elastic bandage in place for 18 to 24 hours, removing it only to apply ice. Elastic bandages that are 2 or 3 inches wide work best for children.

DO NOT

- wrap a compression bandage too tightly.
- allow a child to continue using the injured body part.
- begin wrapping an elastic bandage above the injured area between the injury and the heart, because this can significantly reduce blood flow to the entire limb. Instead, begin wrapping below the injury to provide compression without restricting blood flow.

4. **Elevation.** Elevate the injury above the level of the heart by placing the injured limb on several pillows. This allows gravity to aid in limiting blood flow to the injury and reducing the swelling.

5. You might need to make arrangements for the child to have an x-ray, if there is severe pain or significant swelling.

6. Call the child's parent.

Bruises

Bruises often accompany the interactions of active children, especially those that engage in vigorous play. Bruises occur when small blood vessels and other cells break open underneath the skin and bleed into muscles and other soft tissue. Initially, a bruised area is red and swollen and then gradually turns blue or purple. As the blood is absorbed over the next few days, the area turns yellow and fades as it heals.

What to Do

1. Apply ice or a cold pack wrapped in a wet cloth against the skin.

2. Elevate the arm or leg if the bruise is large and if you do not suspect a broken bone. If the bruise is unusually swollen or painful, the bone under the bruise might be broken. Notify the child's parent.

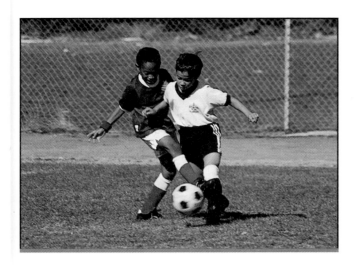

Sports-Related Injuries*

Children as young as age 4 participate in organized sports, both individual and team. The pressure from coaches and parents to excel and to win, not just to participate for fun, can be enormous. Many injuries can be attributed to repetitive overuse or cross training, which can result in sprains, torn muscles and cartilage, inflamed tendons and joints, and stress fractures.

It is estimated that 4 million children seek treatment in hospital emergency rooms every year as a result of sports-related injuries and that another 8 million are treated by health care providers for these injuries.

Following these guidelines when children participate in organized sporting activities might help to prevent an injury.

- The individual who is responsible for coaching a sport should have experience, training, and education in the health risks of training children too vigorously.

- All coaches, whether paid or volunteer, should be trained in first aid.

- Children should have a complete physical examination before participating in sports activities.

- Children should know what safety equipment is necessary, and it should be available to them consistently. Equipment should fit properly.

- Playing areas should be free of hazardous debris and regraded when necessary.

- Time should be included for warm-up and cool-down activities.

- Pain is an indication that something is wrong. Children should never be told to "work through it."

*Adapted from Sports and Injuries, The National Youth Sports Foundation for the Prevention of Athletic Injuries, Inc.

STUDY QUESTIONS 8

Name _____ Course _____ Date _____

1. Circle true (T) or false (F) for the following statements about fractures.

   T   F   a. Fractures in children are worrisome, because damage to the growth plate can cause shortening of the bone.

   T   F   b. Fractures only damage bones.

   T   F   c. Ice is effective in controlling swelling in a fracture.

   T   F   d. The bone is always visible in an open fracture.

2. Which of the following are signs or symptoms of a fractured bone? Circle yes (Y) or no (N).

   Y   N   a. Pain and tenderness

   Y   N   b. Vomiting

   Y   N   c. Swelling

   Y   N   d. Deformity

   Y   N   e. Loss of mobility

   Y   N   f. Fever

3. Five-year-old Kim screams in pain after leaping from a swing. He is huddled on the ground holding his arm. He tells you it hurts so much he doesn't want you to touch it. You suspect that he has fractured his arm. Circle yes (Y) or no (N) for the following first aid actions.

   Y   N   a. Gently remove the clothing surrounding the injury.

   Y   N   b. Place ice or a cold pack directly over the injury.

   Y   N   c. Offer him a cool drink.

   Y   N   d. Immobilize his arm in the position in which he is most comfortable.

4. Simon twists his ankle while racing a friend to the swing set. You suspect that he has sprained it. What first aid measures do you take for this soft tissue injury?

   a. _____

   b. _____

   c. _____

   d. _____

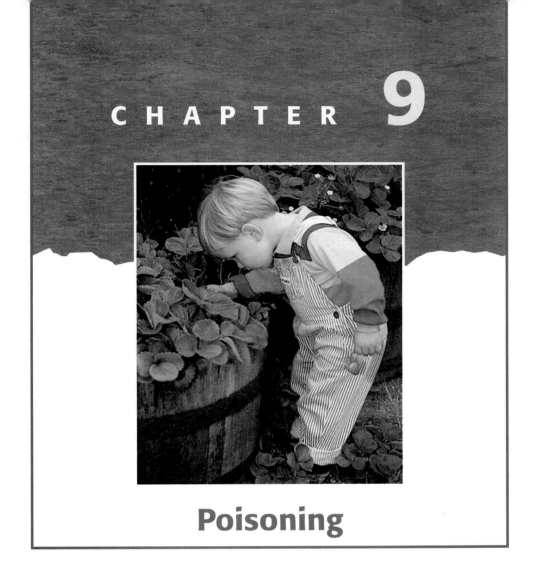

CHAPTER 9

Poisoning

A poison is a substance that when swallowed, inhaled, absorbed through the skin (as from a plant), or injected (as from an insect sting) can cause illness, damage, and sometimes death. Often, exposure to only a tiny amount can have serious consequences.

Poisoning is one of the most common emergencies in children under the age of 5. It almost always happens in a home. Swallowed poisons account for most of these emergencies. Fortunately, the incidence of swallowed poisoning has decreased in the last two decades because the improved packaging of many poisonous substances makes it more difficult for children to open the containers. Also, access to proper treatment through regional poison control centers and greater public awareness of poison prevention methods have helped to reduce the number and the severity of accidental poisonings.

However, poisonings still remain a major reason for emergency care and hospital admissions. For every poisoning death among children under age 5, there are 80,000 to 90,000 other children who receive emergency medical treatment and 20,000 who need hospitalization. Fortunately, approximately three quarters of all poisonings can be successfully treated where they occur.

Swallowed Poisons

Any substance that a child swallows can cause harm in a large enough dose. Many of the products we use every day to clean our homes, treat our illnesses, maintain our yards, and pursue our hobbies are highly toxic and potentially fatal. They can have tragic consequences when swallowed. In general, the poisonous substances that are the most devastating to children are medications, cleaning products, pesticides, alcoholic beverages, and petroleum products, such as gasoline.

Preventing a Swallowed Poisoning

Young children are curious by nature. Colored plastic containers, colorful pills, and never-before-seen items invite the child to explore. Taste is the first sense toddlers and many preschoolers use when investigating something new, regardless of whether it is a toy, food, chemical, or plant. Accidental poisonings often happen when adults are tired or preoccupied, when children have been left alone (even momentarily), and when proper storage or disposal of a poison is either interrupted or forgotten. Most accidental childhood poisonings can be prevented by safe use and proper storage of household products and medicines. Storing chemicals correctly takes only a few moments, but coping with the consequences of swallowed poison can take a very long time.

Safety recommendations for avoiding a swallowed poisoning include:

1. Eliminate careless storage of poisons. Keep all chemical substances, including household products and all chemicals kept in the garage and basement, out of the reach of children. Store them in locked cabinets or on high shelves. Lock medicine cabinets. Purchase corrosive chemicals, such as drain cleaner, in single-use quantities whenever possible.

Some Common Household Poisons

Acetaminophen	Ibuprofen
Aftershave lotion	Insecticides
Alcohol rub	Kerosene
Alcoholic beverages	Laundry detergents
Ammonia	Lighter fluid
Antifreeze	Lime
Antihistamines	Lye
Aspirin	Matches
Bathroom cleaning products	Mothballs
	Mouthwash
Bleach, liquid or powder	Nail polish
	Oven cleaners
Boric acid	Paintbrush cleaners
Button-size batteries	Paint removers
Charcoal lighter fluid	Perfume
Corn and wart remover	Plants and plant food
	Plastic and rubber cements
Cosmetics	
Deodorant	Rug cleaners
Diabetic urine test tablets	Rust remover
	Scouring powder
Dishwasher powders	Shampoo
Dishwashing liquids	Shoe polish
Drain cleaners	Silver polish
Fabric softeners	Spot removers
Fireworks	Sunscreen products
Flea powder	Tobacco
Floor and furniture waxes and polishes	Toilet cleaners
	Turpentine
Gasoline	Varnish
Grease remover	Weight reduction pills
Hair dyes and permanents	Windshield washer fluid
Hair straighteners	
Hydrogen peroxide	Wood preservatives

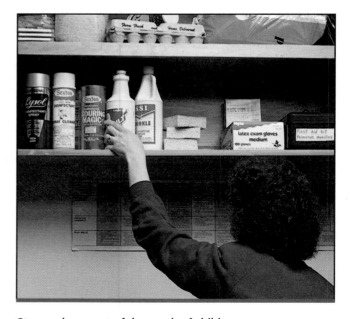

Store poisons out of the reach of children.

2. Conduct a child's eye–level inspection of every room in your child care center or home to see what dangers you can find.

3. Avoid interruption when using a poisonous product. If you must leave your work area, put the chemical safely away or carry it with you.

4. Do not store household products with food; the differences between them might not be apparent to a young child.

5. Purchase products with child-resistant safety caps whenever possible. Although much safer, these containers are not completely child-proof. Children watch and imitate adult behavior and some children can master the task of getting the lids off. Also, the lids do not work unless they are completely closed. Accidental poisonings commonly occur with vitamins and acetaminophen, both of which come in child-resistant containers.

6. Be careful with the storage of products, such as cosmetics and hair and body care items. They do not come in child-resistant packaging but are poisons just the same.

7. Keep products in their original, labeled containers. If a poisonous substance is swallowed, correct identification is critical for proper emergency treatment. Do not reuse empty containers, such as soft drink bottles, juice bottles, paper cups, and empty food containers.

What Poisons Children

Nearly three quarters of the reported exposures to poisons involve products and substances found in the following nine categories:

Medicines and vitamins	25.8%
Cleaning substances and chemicals	13.1%
Cosmetics and personal care products	8.5%
Plants	5.4%
Bites and envenomization	4.3%
Insecticides/pesticides	4.1%
Foreign objects	3.7%
Hydrocarbons*	3.4%
Alcoholic beverages	2.6%

*Such as gasoline and kerosene.

Adapted from American Association of Poison Control Centers.

The #1 Poison

The single most common poison exposure in young children is acetaminophen, a medicine common in almost every home, but especially in those with children. It is used as a fever reducer and pain reliever. The accidental overdoses often occur because parents are not aware that the infant acetaminophen and the toddler acetaminophen differ in strength, and the adult fails to follow the directions on the bottle. The infant product is actually stronger than the toddler product, because it is intended to be given in a very small amount from a dropper. If an adult gives the infant liquid to an older child, using a medicine spoon or kitchen measuring spoon, the child receives too much acetaminophen. Such a tiny mistake can have a powerful effect, especially on the child's liver. Parents of young children are urged to consult their child's health care provider concerning which acetaminophen product and strength to give.

8. To avoid accidental poisonings with medicines, follow these rules:

- Keep medicines in a locked cabinet. Never keep medicines on a bedside table or in a drawer.

- Remember that nonprescription medicines are not less dangerous than prescription medicines. Both can be deadly.

- Give prescription medicine only to the child for whom it is intended. What is helpful for one child can harm another.

- Check the medicine label for the dosage each time you give it. The wrong dose of medicine can poison a child. More is not better when giving medicine. Use a dose-measuring cup or spoon.

- Only one adult in a child care center should be responsible for administering a child's medicine, so that the child does not accidentally receive more than one dose.

- Never call medicine "candy" in an effort to get a child to swallow it. This practice invites a later poisoning accident.

- Flush old medicine down the toilet, and rinse out the container before discarding it.

9. Look for poison hazards when taking a young child on a field trip or into a home or other

building where poison prevention steps might be inadequate.

10. Keep all pocketbooks out of the reach of children.

11. Plants can also contain potentially dangerous chemicals. These rules apply to plants:

    - Identify all of the indoor and outdoor plants at your child care center or home. If possible, move poisonous plants out of the reach of children. Refer to the *Poisonous Plants* section in this chapter for information on nonpoisonous plants to use in and around the center or home.

    - Avoid decorating your center or home with the December holiday plants, including poinsettia, holly, mistletoe, boxwood, bittersweet, Christmas rose, and Christmas cherry. Although festive, all are dangerous and some are extremely poisonous.

    - When outdoors, teach children to keep all plants, including flowers and berries, out of their mouths. Do not share your knowledge of edible wild plants with young children, because they are not always able to correctly identify safe plants when you are not around.

    - Store plant food with other poisons.

12. Be sure that the art product packages in your child care center are labeled "AP" for approved product or "CP" for certified product. Some art supplies can be toxic if ingested or inhaled. See *Art Materials: Recommendations for Children under 12.*

13. Be sure that all lead paint has been removed from your child care center or home. See *Lead Poisoning in Children,* Chapter 17.

Be Prepared!

Maintaining good poison prevention habits includes being prepared for a poisoning. Taking the following precautions now will prepare you to respond quickly and appropriately if a poisoning ever occurs in your center or home.

- Keep the telephone number of your local poison control center and rescue ambulance posted at every telephone in your child care center or home.

- Keep syrup of ipecac in the first aid kit or other handy location, out of children's reach. Ipecac is a plant extract that, when swallowed, is the fastest and most effective way to cause vomiting.

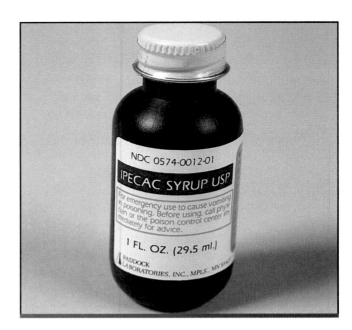

Syrup of ipecac

When Poisonings Occur

Poisonings occur throughout the day, but the peak hours for poisoning incidents are between 5:00 PM and 9:00 PM.

It is available without a prescription. It is important to know that ipecac is used *only* to treat swallowed poisons that can be vomited safely; with other swallowed poisons, its use can be devastating. *Never* give it until the poison control center tells you to do so. Check the expiration date on your bottle of syrup of ipecac.

- Call your local poison control center whenever you have a question about a medicine, household chemical, or plant.

What to Look For

The signs that the child exhibits depend on the chemical swallowed and the amount of time that has passed. After a poison is swallowed, absorption can begin in as little as a few minutes, making immediate action necessary.

Early signs include:

- Opened container of medicine or chemical kept in the household or garage

- Unusual odors from mouth or stains on skin or clothes
- Sudden changes in behavior, including fear, irritability, or overactivity
- Painful burns in and around the mouth that indicate that the child has come in contact with a corrosive chemical
- Nausea, vomiting

  Later signs include:

- Headache
- Cold, clammy skin
- Abdominal pain or cramping
- Weakness and disorientation
- Slurred speech
- Breathing difficulties
- Drowsiness
- Seizures
- Unconsciousness

What to Do

1. Remove any pills, crystals, or other traces of poison from the child's mouth.
2. Gather information. Remain calm. Ask questions in a nonaccusatory manner to help coax some important answers from the child. However, do not delay calling the poison control center if you do not have precise information for every point. Try to determine the following:
   - Age and approximate weight of the child
   - Name or type of chemical swallowed
   - Amount swallowed, such as: "just a sip," "half of the pills," "all of the liquid"
   - How long ago
   - Child's condition, such as: conscious, vomiting, burned mouth, abdominal pain
3. If the child swallowed a *corrosive chemical* (one that burns and causes considerable pain), give immediately ½ to ¾ of a cup (4 to 6 ounces), but no more, of milk or cold water. This amount rinses the poison from the mouth and throat but is not enough to cause vomiting. See *Corrosive Chemicals: A Red Alert.*
4. Call your local poison control center. Have the child and the container with you when you make the call. Follow their instructions.
5. If the child is drowsy or unresponsive or may vomit or has swallowed a corrosive chemical, place the child in the recovery position on the left side. Lying on the left side slows the emptying of the stomach contents, increasing the chance of the poisoning being successfully treated. Once the poison passes from the stomach into the small intestine, it is absorbed into the bloodstream. This position also keeps

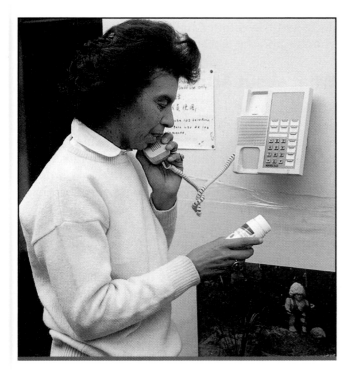

If a child swallows a poisonous substance, call your local poison control center immediately.

Corrosive Chemicals: A Red Alert

Swallowing any chemical can have serious consequences, but swallowing a corrosive chemical has additional dangers. Besides the potentially life-threatening consequences of such a destructive poison in the body, the act of swallowing it can cause severe burns and pain to the lips, mouth, throat, stomach, and small intestine. These corrosive chemicals should not be intentionally vomited through the use of syrup of ipecac, because the throat and mouth will be damaged further if exposed to the chemical again. A child who has swallowed a corrosive substance must be treated in an emergency medical facility immediately. This is a life-threatening emergency.

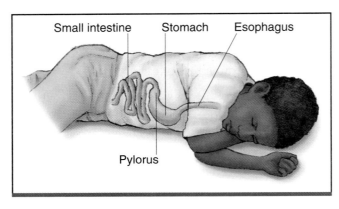

The left side-lying position slows the emptying of the stomach.

DO NOT

- **waste time calling a pharmacist, hospital emergency department, or physician when a poisoning occurs. Call the poison control center for the most accurate first aid advice.**
- **follow directions on the product container. Neither the directions nor suggested antidotes are as safe or effective as contacting your poison control center immediately.**
- **give syrup of ipecac to induce vomiting unless told to do so by the poison control center.**
- **give syrup of ipecac to induce vomiting if the child is drowsy, unresponsive, or seizing. The child might choke or vomit might enter lungs.**
- **give milk or water to dilute a swallowed poison unless told to do so by the poison control center. This may cause some chemicals to dissolve more quickly and move into the small intestine, where absorption into the bloodstream takes place.**
- **use old-fashioned remedies, such as swallowing salt water or sticking a spoon or fingers in the back of the throat, as your first choice to induce vomiting. If vomiting occurs, it will not be of the volume that ipecac produces.**
- **give syrup of ipecac to induce vomiting if there are burns or blisters present from a corrosive chemical in and around the mouth. Vomiting a corrosive chemical causes even more tissue damage, because the skin is exposed to the chemical a second time.**
- **attempt to give activated charcoal in the child care center or home. See *What About Activated Charcoal?* If indicated in the treatment of a poisoning, it is best administered in an emergency medical facility. Do not give it along with syrup of ipecac.**

the airway open and, if vomiting occurs, allows it to drain from the mouth.

6. Send someone to call for emergency medical help, if needed.
7. Monitor the ABCDs and treat accordingly.
8. Call the child's parent.

What If the Poison Control Center Tells You to Give Ipecac?

Most swallowed poisons are noncorrosive and do not burn the tissue of the mouth and throat but can cause damage if absorbed by the body. The most effective way to rid the body of most of a noncorrosive poison is by vomiting promptly. Sometimes the body does this on its own, but it can also be accomplished by having the child swallow syrup of ipecac, a plant extract that causes vomiting. However, ipecac is given *only* under the direction of the poison control center. The staff will know how much to give and what fluids the child can drink. It should be given within 30 minutes after the poisoning. Additional fluids in the stomach, as well as walking or other movement, speed the action of the ipecac. Most children vomit within 15 to 20 minutes. This will remove a large amount, but not all, of the poison in the stomach.

The poison control center staff will know if the child needs further medical attention. If the child does, and has vomited, take a sample of the vomitus and the labeled poison container with you.

What about Activated Charcoal?

Activated charcoal is very effective in treating a great many poisons but is seldom given to a child in a child care center or in a home, because it is difficult to administer and is not effective for every poison. In the stomach, activated charcoal binds with the poison, preventing it from being absorbed into the bloodstream while traveling through the digestive system. In an emergency medical facility, it is often given after treatment with ipecac for more dangerous poisonings because vomiting induced by ipecac does not remove all of the poison. It should not be given at the same time as ipecac, because it can bind the ipecac and prevent vomiting.

Activated charcoal comes pre-mixed or as a powder to mix with water, which forms a chalky, milkshake-like drink that resembles black mud. When minutes count, convincing a frightened young child to swallow a large amount of this thick liquid is more than most parents or child care providers can manage. Activated charcoal is best given in an emergency medical facility, where it can be administered through a tube much more easily than by drinking. In addition, if the poisoning emergency is such that activated charcoal is needed, it is wise to be in a medical facility where observation and further treatment can be provided.

Poison control centers rarely recommend that activated charcoal be given to a child outside of a medical setting. Nonetheless, if your child care center or home is a long distance from emergency medical help, you may want to check with your local poison control center for their recommendations about having activated charcoal available.

Poison Control Centers: A Life Saver

Poison control centers can provide help for every kind of poisoning and are the most reliable source of information about poisons. These centers are located throughout the United States and are staffed by experts who have special training in toxicology, the study of poisons. They have access to detailed product information on hundreds of thousands of household products and medications. They also have access to a network of specialists with information about such uncommon poisons as mushrooms and snake venom. In addition, poison control centers have a variety of informative pamphlets to help you prevent an accidental poisoning.

Poison control centers serve emergency medical facilities, community health care providers, and the general public. They are equipped to answer routine questions and to handle poisoning emergencies. They can determine whether a poisoning can be treated over the telephone or whether the child needs to be seen in an emergency medical facility. If the poisoning can be treated at home, they provide specific directions on what steps to take. In addition, they can help arrange for emergency medical transportation, if necessary.

Everyone in the United States can reach a regional poison control center with either a local phone call or by using an "800" number. Check your telephone book or call telephone information to obtain the number for the poison control center in your area. This number should be posted next to each telephone in your child care center or home.

Poisonous Plants

Like many adults, most young children know little about toxic plants and cannot be relied upon to recognize them. Because many toddlers and preschooolers use their senses of touch and taste when investigating something new, it is not unusual for children to touch and mouth leaves, berries, and flowers. Poisonings can occur from swallowing a plant, absorbing a toxin through the skin, or inhaling fumes from a fire that contains a poisonous plant. Some poisonous plants cause only minor stomach irritation; others can cause abdominal cramping, breathing difficulties, and even death. There are many poisonous plants and no "sure-fire" way to tell a poisonous one from a nonpoisonous one. See the safety recommendations concerning plants earlier in this chapter.

Swallowed Plants

What to Do

If a child in your care swallows any part of a plant, take the child and a sample of the plant to the telephone and call the poison control center. They will tell you what to do.

For the safety of the children in your care, learn the names of the plants, trees, and shrubbery growing on the property where your child care center or home is located. Also learn whether they are poisonous plants or plants that are generally recognized as safe. If a child swallows a part of a plant that is considered safe, it is best to call the poison control center and discuss the situation with them.

Poison Ivy, Poison Oak, and Poison Sumac

A small number of plants cause an allergic reaction when they make contact with skin. The best known are poison ivy, poison oak, and poison sumac, all of which are found throughout the United States. Exposure to the oil of these plants can cause a delayed allergic reaction in the form of a rash that varies in severity. A child can be exposed to the oil of these plants directly by touching the leaves, stems, or roots or indirectly by touching exposed tools, clothes, pets, or any other article touched by the plant. Smoke from a brush fire containing the burning plant will carry this oil in tiny droplets to the skin and into the nose, throat, and lungs. Contact with these plants can happen during any

Art Materials: Recommendations for Children under 12

Do Not Use	Substitutes
Dusts and Powders	
1. Clay in dry form. Powdered clay, which is easily inhaled, contains free silica and possibly asbestos. Do not sand dry clay pieces or do other dust-producing activities.	1. Order talc-free premixed clay (e.g., Amaco white clay). Wet mop or sponge surfaces thoroughly after using clay.
2. Ceramic glazes or copper enamels.	2. Use water-based paints instead of glazes. Artwork may be waterproofed with acrylic-based mediums.
3. Cold water dyes, fiber-reactive dyes, or other commercial dyes.	3. Use vegetable and plant dyes (e.g., onionskins, tea, flowers) and food dyes.
4. Instant papier mâché (creates inhalable dust and some may contain asbestos, fibers, lead from pigments in colored printing inks, etc.).	4. Make papier mâché from black and white newspaper and library or white paste, or use approved papier mâché.
5. Powdered tempera colors (create inhalable dusts and some tempera colors contain toxic pigments, preservatives, etc.).	5. Use liquid paints or paints the teacher premixes.
6. Pastels, chalks, or dry markers that create dust.	6. Use crayons, oil pastels, or dustless chalks.
Solvents	
1. Solvents (e.g., turpentine, shellac, toluene, rubber cement thinner) and solvent-containing materials (solvent-based inks, alkyd paints, rubber cement).	1. Use water-based products only.
2. Solvent-based silk screen and other printing inks.	2. Use water-based silk screen inks, block printing or stencil inks containing safe pigments.
3. Aerosol sprays.	3. Use water-based paints with brushes or spatter techniques.
4. Epoxy, instant glue, airplane glue, or other solvent-based adhesives.	4. Use white glue, school paste, and preservative-free wheat paste.
5. Permanent felt tip markers, which may contain toluene or other toxic solvents.	5. Use only water-based markers.
Toxic Metals	
1. Stained glass projects using lead came, solder, flux, etc.	1. Use colored cellophane and black paper to simulate lead.
2. Arsenic, cadmium, chrome, mercury, lead, manganese, or other toxic metals, which may occur in pigments, metal filings, metal enamels, ceramic glazes, metal casting, etc.	2. Use approved materials only.
Miscellaneous	
1. Photographic chemicals.	1. Use blueprint paper and make sun grams, or use Polaroid cameras.
2. Casting plaster. Creates dust and casting hands and body parts has resulted in serious burns.	2. Teacher can mix plaster in a separate ventilated area or outdoors for plaster casting.
3. Acid etches and pickling baths.	3. No acceptable substitutes. Should not use techniques employing these chemicals.
4. Scented felt-tip markers. These teach children bad habits about eating and sniffing art materials.	4. Use water-based markers.

This information was excerpted from The Center for Safety in the Art's Datasheet, *Children's Art Supplies Can Be Toxic*. Further information is available from Art Hazards Information Center, 5 Beekman Street, New York, NY 10038.

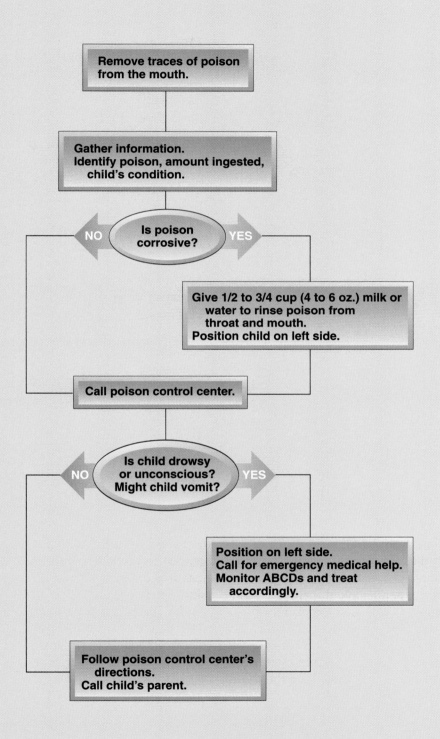

Remove traces of poison from the mouth.

Gather information. Identify poison, amount ingested, child's condition.

Is poison corrosive?

NO — YES

Give 1/2 to 3/4 cup (4 to 6 oz.) milk or water to rinse poison from throat and mouth. Position child on left side.

Call poison control center.

Is child drowsy or unconscious? Might child vomit?

NO — YES

Position on left side. Call for emergency medical help. Monitor ABCDs and treat accordingly.

Follow poison control center's directions. Call child's parent.

Poisonous Plants

The following list provides the names of some of the more common indoor and outdoor poisonous plants. Though the toxicity varies, ingesting or swallowing any amount of these plants is dangerous.

A
Acorn
Aloe vera
Amaryllis
Anthurium
Arrowhead
Autumn crocus
Avocado leaves
Azalea
B
Baneberry
Belladonna
Bird-of-paradise
Bittersweet
Black locust
Bleeding heart
Boston ivy
Boxwood
Buckeye
Buttercup
C
Caladium
Calla lily
Caper spurge
Carnation
Castor bean

China berry
Chrysanthemum
Crown of thorns
Cyclamen
D
Daffodil bulb
Daisy
Daphne
Delphinium
Dieffenbachia
Dumb cane
E
Elephant ear
English ivy
Eucalyptus
F
Four o'clock
Foxglove
G
Glory lily
Golden chain tree
Ground ivy
H
Holly
Hyacinth
Hydrangea

I
Iris
J
Jack-in-the-pulpit
Jerusalem cherry
Jessamine
Jimson weed (thorn apple)
Juniper
L
Lantana
Larkspur
M
Marijuana
Mistletoe
Morning glory
Mountain laurel
Mushrooms
N
Narcissus
Nightshade
O
Ohio buckeye
Oleander
P
Periwinkle
Philodendron

Pits of apricot, cherry, peach, and plum
Poinsettia
Poison hemlock
Poison ivy
Poison oak
Poison sumac
Privet
R
Rhododendron
Rhubarb leaves
Rubber vine
S
Shamrocks
Skunk cabbage
Sweet pea
T
Tobacco
Tomato leaves
Tulip bulbs
W
Water hemlock
Wisteria
Yew

season of the year and from handling any part of the plant—not just the leaves.

Unfortunately most people cannot recognize these plants so they can neither avoid them nor wash and rinse the skin immediately after exposure, which sometimes lessens the reaction. To help everyone avoid these plants, teach the children in your care to watch out for plants that are characterized by leaves growing in groups of threes and teach them the short rhyme, "Leaves of three—LET THEM BE!"

What to Look For

Poison ivy, poison oak, and poison sumac rashes can vary from a mild case with itching and redness to a severe case that also includes blisters and a generalized swelling of the area. Sometimes a severe rash is accompanied by a secondary infection of the skin, causing the infected area to be extremely tender and to appear yellow from pus accumulation. It commonly takes 1 or 2 days for symptoms of contact with these plants to appear.

What to Do

1. If you suspect that a child in your care was exposed to one of these plants, immediately wash the area with soap and flush with plenty of running water to rinse the plant oil off. Most importantly, the area needs to be rinsed well.

Nonpoisonous Plants

The following plants are generally considered to be nontoxic. However, it is always possible for an individual to have an allergic reaction from ingesting a part of one of these plants.

African violet
Aluminum plant
Asparagus fern
Baby's breath or baby's tears
Bachelor buttons
Begonia
Boston fern
Cacti (certain varieties)
Christmas cactus
Coleus
Corn plant
Crape myrtle
Creeping Jenny
Crocus
Dahlia
Dandelion
Dogwood
Dracaena
Easter lily
Forget-me-not
Forsythia
Fuschia
Gardenia
Geranium
Gloxinia
Hibiscus
Honeysuckle
Hoya
Impatiens
Jade plant

Kalanchoe
Lipstick plant
Monkey plant
Norfolk pine
Orchid
Pansy
Petunia
Phlox
Prayer plant
Purple passion
Rose
Rubber plant
Sedum
Sensitive plant
Snapdragon
Spider plant
Swedish ivy
Tiger lily
Umbrella plant
Umbrella tree
Venus flytrap
Violet
Wandering Jew
Wax plant
Weeping fig
Weeping willow
Yucca
Zebra plant
Zinnia

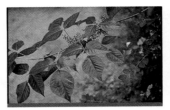

Poison ivy

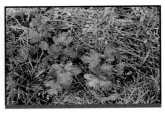

Poison oak

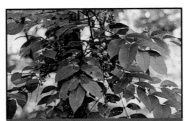

Poison sumac

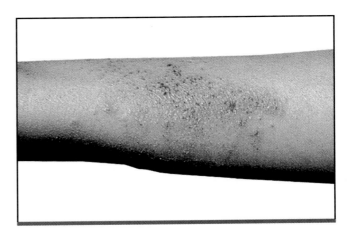

Poison ivy rash

Sometimes the severity of the rash can be lessened if the soaping and rinsing occurs within the first few minutes after exposure.

2. Notify the parent at the end of the day about the exposure and treatment. Should the child have a moderate to severe reaction including intense itching, burning, and general discomfort, a few days at home would be appropriate.

DO NOT

- touch or rub the area if you suspect contact with poison ivy, poison oak, or poison sumac, because the oil can be spread all over the body and from person to person in this way.
- put the child in a bathtub of water after the exposure in an attempt to remove the oil, because this spreads the oil to other parts of the body.
- wipe with pretreated towelettes, because they are not effective in removing the oil, and wiping back and forth or in a circular motion spreads the oil.
- apply lotions to moisturize skin.

Home Care Treatment

Once the rash develops, a parent at home can use any or all of the following suggestions for trying to relieve the symptoms.

1. To relieve itching:

   - The affected area can be placed in very warm water. The water should be hot enough to make the skin pink, but not hot enough to burn. This helps the cells release the substance that causes itching and gives the child several hours of relief.

   - Baking soda can be used as often as necessary either in a bath or as a paste of one teaspoon of water to three teaspoons of baking soda . This temporarily reduces itching and burning. A bath with 1 to 2 cups of a colloid oatmeal, such as Aveeno, also helps with discomfort. Be careful, because the oatmeal makes the tub slippery.

   - Calamine lotion can reduce itching and can promote drying of the blistered area.

2. Cortisone medicines in strengths suggested or prescribed by the child's health care provider can speed the healing of a moderate to severe rash. Antibiotics might be prescribed if the area becomes infected.

3. Trimming fingernails short, scrubbing them with a nail brush, and discouraging scratching reduces the risk of infection and of further irritation to the skin.

4. To contain the spread of poison ivy rash, wash in detergent and hot water all clothing that might have come in contact with the plant. If the child is known to have a severe reaction to poison ivy, poison oak, or poison sumac, wash the clothing twice. Also wash everything that accompanied the child, including shoes, toys, tools, and pets. The oil remains potent and can continue to spread for weeks to unsuspecting people who touch these items in the area where the oil adheres.

If the child has a moderate to severe reaction, it is possible that he or she will be at home and unable to attend school or child care for a few days.

A child can return to your child care center or home when feeling better, as long as the affected areas are covered with a nonstick dressing. This prevents you or other children from coming in contact with the fluid they contain and protects the child's rash from becoming infected. The breaking and weeping blisters do not contain the plant oil that causes the skin reaction. Contact with these weeping blisters cannot spread the poison ivy rash to others. Be certain that all staff know this often-misunderstood fact.

Inhaled Poisons

Poisoning by inhalation can occur dramatically, as in smoke inhalation during a building fire. It can also occur insidiously, as in carbon monoxide poisoning from a faulty furnace, a kerosene space heater, or a car with the motor running in an enclosed garage. Sadly, it can also occur when a child experiments with intentionally inhaling a chemical, such as the fumes from rubber cement and model glue.

While the presence of flames brings the ultimate urgency to remove people from a burning structure, it is the smoke and fumes from the burning building that are the most deadly. Toxins can be absorbed, and irritation or chemical burns of the airway and lungs can cause swelling hours after the exposure.

Inhalation Injuries and Older Children

Sometimes older children experiment with inhaling solvents in products such as model glue, white correction fluid, or rubber cement, or they spray various aerosols from cans directly into the nose in the hopes of "getting high." Although this can be a part of a larger drug addiction problem, sometimes it is the only substance abuse activity in which a child experiments. For some, it is part of the normal inquisitiveness about the forbidden at this age. What must be understood, however, is that intentionally inhaling fumes is extremely dangerous.

The immediate signs and symptoms of an acute overdose of an inhaled toxin can include headache, nausea, loss of coordination and judgment, coughing and sneezing, and nosebleed. Deeply inhaling a large amount of vapor over a short time can cause disorientation, violent behavior, unconsciousness, slowed breathing and heart rate, or even respiratory and cardiac arrest. Eventually, repeated abuse can permanently damage the liver and the nervous system. Elementary school–aged children must be taught the dangers of inhaling these vapors to avoid choosing this type of recreational activity in their preteen and teenage years.

POISON IVY, POISON OAK, AND POISON SUMAC

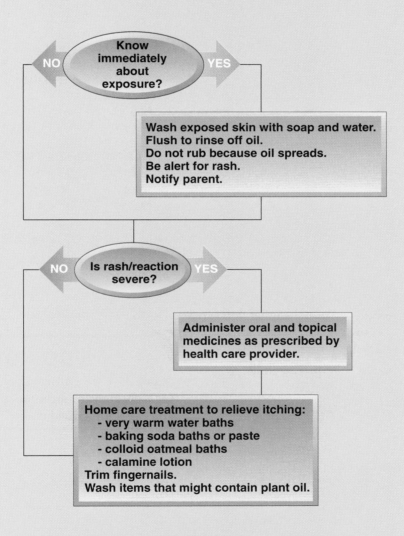

Know immediately about exposure?

NO — YES

Wash exposed skin with soap and water.
Flush to rinse off oil.
Do not rub because oil spreads.
Be alert for rash.
Notify parent.

Is rash/reaction severe?

NO — YES

Administer oral and topical medicines as prescribed by health care provider.

Home care treatment to relieve itching:
- **very warm water baths**
- **baking soda baths or paste**
- **colloid oatmeal baths**
- **calamine lotion**
Trim fingernails.
Wash items that might contain plant oil.

In other, less dramatic, cases of inhaled poisoning, it might be difficult to tell that a child was exposed to a toxic chemical. A child's complaint of feeling sick or having the "flu" could be a signal of an inhaled poisoning. However, an inhaled poison will not produce the fever, aching muscles, or enlarged lymph nodes that the "flu" or similar viral infection does. A building-wide poisoning, such as carbon monoxide, affects everyone in the building, including family pets.

What to Look For

- Headache
- Nausea, vomiting
- Blurred vision
- Ringing in the ears
- Dizziness and confusion
- Muscular weakness
- Seizures
- Chest pain
- Difficulty breathing
- Unconsciousness
- Respiratory and cardiac arrest

What to Do

1. Remove the child from the toxic area or product. Be certain that all people are out. Get help from fire and rescue personnel so that you do not jeopardize your own health or safety in trying to get others away from toxic fumes.
2. Call for emergency medical help. The child might need 100% oxygen.
3. Check and monitor the child's ABCDs and treat accordingly.

Not a Place for Children

Allowing children to ride in the enclosed back of a pickup truck is dangerous, not only because they are not properly restrained, but because they can be exposed to dangerous levels of carbon monoxide. Truck exhaust fumes leak into the enclosed space and accumulate because the ventilation is poor. Because carbon monoxide is odorless, there is no warning that poisonous fumes are building up. Unfortunately, some children have died and others have been left with permanent brain damage from breathing carbon monoxide fumes while riding in this area. Several states have already outlawed riding in the back of an enclosed pickup truck. The only safe way to transport children in this type of vehicle is in the passenger areas of the cab.

4. If the child is unresponsive but breathing, position the child on the left side in the recovery position. This keeps the airway open and is the safest position for vomiting.
5. Seek medical attention even if the child appears to be fully recovered after the exposure to smoke or fumes. Internal damage and toxic effects are often not apparent until several hours later.
6. Notify the child's parent.

DO NOT

- depend on the information on a product label for treatment of an inhaled poisoning. Seek emergency medical care.

Carbon monoxide (CO) is a poisonous gas that is deadly if inhaled in sufficient quantities for enough time. Dangerous concentrations of CO can occur anytime combustion (burning) takes place in a poorly ventilated area.

When something burns, it gives off a number of gases, including: water vapor, carbon dioxide (CO_2) and carbon monoxide (CO). All fuels used in the home can generate CO, including solid fuels (wood, charcoal, and coal), liquid fuels (kerosene, gasoline, and heating fuel oil), and gas fuels (natural gas and propane.) Even a burning cigarette gives off carbon monoxide. So do fuel-burning engines (such as automobiles and generators). The amount of CO given off depends on how much fuel is burned and how efficiently the burning occurs. The amount of CO formed by any kind of burning can increase greatly if the device is not getting enough air. For this reason, any combustion device used indoors must be properly maintained. Devices that burn large quantities of fuel (such as engines, space heaters, and charcoal grills) should not be used indoors or should only be used with very good ventilation. Even a gas stove and oven can be dangerous if used to heat a room, because, with the oven door left open, a much larger amount of fuel than normal is burned, producing far more CO than the home can naturally ventilate.

To minimize the risk of carbon monoxide poisoning, follow these rules:

1. Be sure that the building's central heating system is properly maintained and inspected regularly by a trained professional. Dryers and water heaters powered by gas should also be inspected.

2. Never use a charcoal grill, hibachi, or gas grill inside the home or garage.

3. Only use a gasoline or kerosene space heater for short periods of time and with a window open to provide adequate ventilation of the CO.

4. Always turn off a gasoline or kerosene space heater before going to bed and never run it in a room where someone else is sleeping.

5. Never use a gas stove or oven to heat the living areas of a home.

6. Always check that burners on a gas stove are turned completely off when finished cooking.

7. Never run a car engine in an attached garage, especially with the garage door closed.

The biggest problem with CO is that it "sneaks up" on its victims. Carbon monoxide is odorless, tasteless, invisible, and does not sting or burn the skin or eyes. There is no warning that it is present. Breathing carbon monoxide in a dangerous amount over a short period of time leads to unconsciousness and death. Even breathing small amounts of it over a long period of time can be equally dangerous, because the effects are cumulative over time.

Carbon monoxide detectors similar to smoke detectors are now available and are easy to install. They sound an alarm if the CO level in the enclosed environment reaches a level that is unsafe. Since carbon monoxide quickly distributes itself fairly evenly within a building, it is recommended that CO detectors be installed on a wall or ceiling of the hallway in sleeping areas. The noise of the alarm awakens those who are sleeping behind a closed bedroom door before the CO seeps in. A CO detector is as important as a smoke alarm in any building.

Name _____ Course _____ Date _____

1. Three-year-old Angela brings you an empty bottle of children's chewable acetaminophen. She has a sweet smell on her breath and you suspect that she swallowed the pills. You take the bottle and the child with you to the phone and you call the poison control center. What information will the poison control center want to know?

   a. _____
   b. _____
   c. _____
   d. _____
   e. _____

2. Who decides whether a swallowed poison must be treated with syrup of ipecac?
   _____

3. Why should syrup of ipecac not be given if there are burns or blisters around the mouth from a swallowed corrosive chemical?
   _____

4. What is your local poison control center's phone number? _____

5. If a child becomes drowsy after swallowing a poison, what should you do and why?
   _____

6. Circle true (T) or false (F) for each of the following statements about swallowed poisonings.

   T F a. Always induce vomiting with syrup of ipecac in a conscious child who swallows a poison.

   T F b. Follow the directions on the poison container to treat a swallowed poison.

   T F c. Give several glasses of water or milk to dilute a poison before calling the poison control center.

   T F d. Activated charcoal given at the same time as syrup of ipecac improves ipecac's ability to empty the poison from the stomach.

   T F e. Never call medicine "candy" to convince a child to swallow it.

   T F f. There is no reliable way to tell a poisonous plant from a nonpoisonous plant.

   T F g. Activated charcoal is commonly used to treat a poisoning at home.

7. Circle yes (Y) or no (N) for each action. After exposure to poison ivy, oak, or sumac, you should:

   Y N a. wash the area immediately with soap and flush with plenty of running water.

   Y N b. wipe the area with pretreated towelettes.

   Y N c. apply calamine lotion to the rash to reduce itching and promote drying.

   Y N d. use baking soda in a bath or as a paste to reduce itching.

   Y N e. use a moisturizing lotion to keep the skin soft if a rash develops.

   Y N f. Warn others that poison ivy, oak, or sumac can spread from coming in contact with open blisters.

8. Circle yes (Y) or no (N) for each statement about inhaled poisonings.

   Y N a. Follow the information on the product label for treatment of an inhaled poisoning.

   Y N b. Remove the child immediately from the toxic area or product.

   Y N c. Toxic effects from an inhaled poisoning are almost always apparent immediately.

   Y N d. If the child is unresponsive, position the child on the left side.

   Y N e. The child might need 100% oxygen.

   Y N f. Carbon monoxide smells similar to natural gas, which helps to identify it.

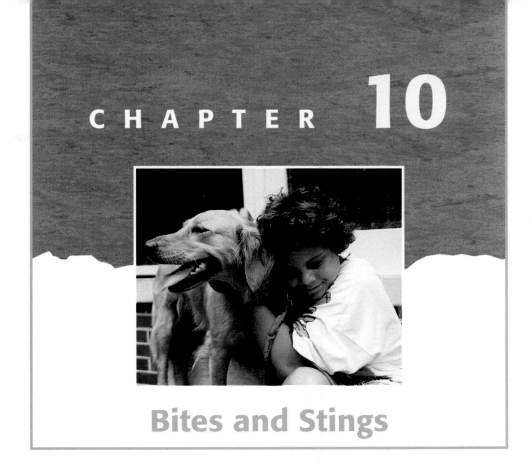

CHAPTER 10

Bites and Stings

Animal Bites

Dogs are responsible for almost 90% of all animal bites in the United States each year. The love and loyalty of dogs, however, make them one of the most popular pets. They can help a child learn to accept responsibility, understand about caring for others, and build self-confidence. Unfortunately, each year there are nearly 1.5 million serious dog bites. It is estimated that over 80% of these injuries involve preschool or school-aged children. Boys are bitten more often than girls, and the majority of these bites are provoked by the child teasing or mistreating the animal. Stray dogs tend to be hesitant around humans and are not involved in biting incidents very often.

Cats are less likely to bite than dogs, but cat bites are more likely to become infected. Wild animals, such as raccoons, skunks, chipmunks, and squirrels, are also known to bite. Any animal bite that breaks the skin can become infected.

The most dangerous infection that can develop after an animal bite is rabies, a viral disease. The rabies virus is present in the saliva of an infected animal and is transmitted to a person through a bite. The disease affects the brain and nervous system. Once rabies symptoms develop, the disease is always fatal. To ensure that this deadly illness does not develop, a person who has been bitten or scratched must be evaluated by a health care provider and receive the rabies vaccine promptly after the bite and complete a series of five injections.

Any warm-blooded animal can carry rabies; however, the animals most commonly infected are raccoons, bats, skunks, foxes, and coyotes. According to the Centers for Disease Control, more than 80% of rabies cases in the United States occur in skunks, raccoons, and bats. A bite from a stray cat or

Cases of Rabies in Animals

37.9%	Skunks
31%	Raccoons
13.5%	Bats
4.1%	Cats
3.9%	Foxes
3.6%	Cattle
2.7%	Dogs
2.1%	Other wild animals
1.3%	Other domestic animals

dog is also of concern, because these animals probably are not immunized. If a child is bitten by one of the animals more commonly infected with rabies, it must be assumed that the animal is rabid.

Small caged animals that are popular in homes and child care centers, such as hamsters, gerbils, and guinea pigs, are generally healthy and do not carry rabies, because they are not exposed to the wild. This is also true for domestic ferrets. Cold-blooded animals do not carry rabies, although bites from such animals as snakes, spiders, and turtles can be dangerous and can become infected.

Many of the animals known to carry rabies are nocturnal. Should you see one of these animals during the day, assume that it is sick, because, otherwise, it would not be wandering at this time. Keep children away from the animal and call the animal control officer in your community to report the animal's location. Do not corner or try to capture the animal yourself.

Until the recent increase in rabid animals in some parts of the United States, household dogs and cats were considered generally rabies-free in many metropolitan areas. But now they are also at risk if they come into contact with a rabid wild animal. It is critical for pet owners to keep their pet's rabies immunization up to date. If you are a dog owner, spay or neuter your dog. Unneutered dogs are three times more likely to bite than neutered dogs are.

If a child is bitten by a domestic cat or dog, parents must check with the animal's owner for verification of the animal's current immunizations. Animal bites that break the skin, however small, introduce bacteria into the blood. Animal bites that do not break the skin are not serious.

What to Do

1. Wear disposable gloves, and use direct pressure and elevation as necessary to control bleeding. If the wound is large or might need stitches, do not attempt to wash the wound.

2. Wash a small wound with soap and water. A small amount of bleeding during washing of the wound helps to remove bacteria from the tissue.

3. Cover the wound with a clean gauze dressing, if needed.

4. Identify the animal that bit the child, if possible. For a cat or dog, check with the owner to be sure that the animal is immunized against rabies.

5. Seek medical attention if the wound is large or if it might need stitches. For smaller bites that break the skin, call the child's parent. Encourage the parent to contact the child's health care provider because of the concern over infection as well as rabies. If the bite does not break the skin, notify the parent at the end of the day.

Observe the wound daily for signs of infection.

Human Bites

Biting occasionally occurs among young children who have not yet learned socially acceptable behavior for expressing themselves and meeting their needs. Fortunately, the urge to bite usually disappears on its own in the course of preschool development.

Many of these bites are minor and more of an emotional upset than a physical injury. However, the human mouth contains a large number of bacteria, some of which can cause infection if introduced into another child's bloodstream through a bite. In fact, the likelihood of infection from a human bite is greater than from an animal bite. Bites that break the skin, however small, introduce bacteria into the blood. Bites that do not break the skin are not serious.

What to Do

1. Wear disposable gloves, and wash the wound with soap and water.

2. Notify the child's parent immediately if a bite breaks the skin. The child's health care provider should be contacted, because the child might

Why Do Dogs Bite?

No matter how obedient and loving dogs can be, they are still animals. Dogs are not usually mean or aggressive, but they will react when threatened or upset or when their hunting instinct is triggered: it is in these situations that dogs are most likely to surprise family or strangers with unexpected aggressiveness or biting.

- Entering a dog's territory, such as its yard, provokes some dogs to become aggressive. Its territory also includes its toys and eating and sleeping areas.
- Running, riding a bike, or kicking a ball past a dog incites a dog's chasing instinct, as does flailing the arms or screaming.
- Pinching, poking, kicking, or other abusive behavior toward the dog causes some dogs to defend themselves in the only way their instinct tells them to.

With these situations in mind, teach children these safety rules about dogs:

- Never mistreat, tease, or make threatening gestures toward a dog.
- Never disturb a dog that is eating or sleeping.
- Adult supervision is necessary when a child feeds a dog.
- Enter a yard where there is a dog only with permission and with the dog's owner accompanying you.
- Do not attempt to get a dog to chase you.
- Never make a quick movement around a dog that might startle or frighten the dog.
- Never break up a dog fight even when one's own dog is involved.
- Avoid strange dogs in the neighborhood, especially if the animal is sick or injured.
- If you are approached by an unfamiliar dog, stop, stand still, and speak softly.

need a tetanus shot or a preventive course of antibiotic medication.

3. If the bite has not broken the skin, notify the child's parent at the end of the day.

Check the wound daily for signs of infection. Read about signs of infection later in this chapter. Repeated biting is unacceptable behavior in a child care center. This behavior should be dealt with promptly to discourage the child from repeated incidents of biting and to protect the other children from injury.

Insect Stings

Bites from such insects as mosquitoes, gnats, fleas, and flies seldom require any medical attention. Stings from the Hymenoptera order of insects, which includes bees, hornets, yellow jackets, polistes (wasps), mud daubers, and ants, are more painful and can even be deadly. When they sting, these insects inject venom that produces a mild local reaction in the majority of the population and, in a small percentage of the population, a more severe allergic reaction. Fortunately, a reaction that is severe enough to cause life-threatening anaphylactic shock happens infrequently. A little less than 1% of the population develops an allergy to this venom, and it is estimated that between 50 and 100

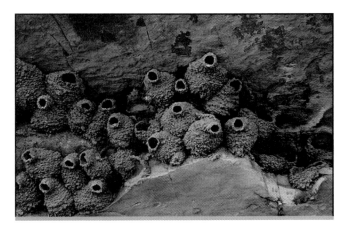

Mud dauber nest

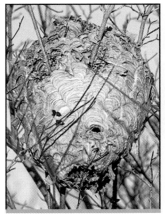

Hornet and yellow jacket nest

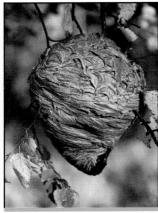

Polistes (wasp) nest

ANIMAL AND HUMAN BITES

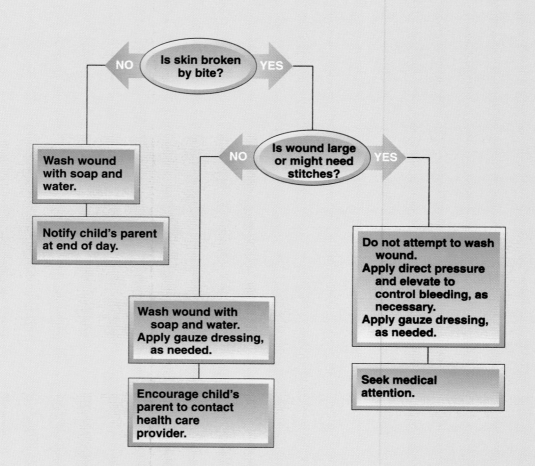

Is skin broken by bite?

NO → Wash wound with soap and water.

Notify child's parent at end of day.

YES → **Is wound large or might need stitches?**

NO → Wash wound with soap and water. Apply gauze dressing, as needed.

Encourage child's parent to contact health care provider.

YES → Do not attempt to wash wound.
Apply direct pressure and elevate to control bleeding, as necessary.
Apply gauze dressing, as needed.

Seek medical attention.

For the child destined to become allergic, the initial sting from an insect of the Hymenoptera order of insects causes the body to produce antibodies that attack the insect venom. This production of antibodies causes no outward sign nor gives any clue that the child will be sensitive to the next sting. However, when the child is stung the next time, the reaction between the insect venom and the antibodies causes many allergic symptoms, the most dangerous of which is swelling in the airway. This makes breathing difficult, if not impossible, and is the cause of death in approximately 75% of the cases in which anaphylactic shock occurs. See *Anaphylaxis,* Chapter 4.

It is important to understand that this allergy to a Hymenoptera sting can develop at any time in life, no matter how many nonallergic stings a person has already had. Initial allergic reactions vary in intensity from person to person, and subsequent stings usually produce increasingly severe symptoms.

Generally, allergic reactions occur immediately or within the first few minutes after the sting. Usually, the earlier the symptoms appear, the more serious the reaction is. Sometimes allergic reactions are slow and worsen over time. This is why it is so important to observe any child for about 30 minutes after any venomous insect sting.

Children who have experienced an allergic reaction of any degree after an insect sting should wear a medical alert necklace stating the allergy to Hymenoptera venom. This immediately identifies the allergy in the event that a rescuer finds the child either experiencing an allergic reaction or unresponsive. After an allergic reaction of any intensity, the child's health care provider should evaluate the child for an allergic self-treatment kit, one of which should be kept with the first aid supplies in your child care center. A school-aged child should keep it on his or her person.

There is treatment available that can reduce an allergic child's sensitivity to the venom. Parents should discuss this with their child's health care provider.

people die every year from a severe allergic reaction to Hymenoptera venom.

What to Look For

A *normal reaction* to an insect sting is a painful surprise to a child but is not serious. This typical reaction lasts up to a few hours and is characterized by immediate stinging pain, redness, mild swelling, and warmth at the site of the sting. Some reactions are more painful, with itching and swelling over a larger area around the sting site, and can last up to a few days. However, these normal reactions are not allergic reactions, because the symptoms remain localized.

An allergic reaction to an insect sting is accompanied by symptoms that affect other areas of the body, including breathing.

Mild allergic reactions are characterized by only a few noticeable signs of allergy, such as mildly flushed skin, a pronounced swelling (especially at the sting site), and hives. Although mild, this degree of reaction is an important warning signal and can occur for up to 24 hours after the sting. The child's parent and health care provider should be contacted. Sometimes the health care provider prescribes a liquid antihistamine to help control

mild symptoms. The antihistamine in the liquid form is easier for a young child to swallow, and it also works more quickly inside the body than taking the pill form of the medicine.

Severe allergic reactions vary in intensity and are very worrisome reactions. An extreme allergy produces anaphylactic shock and usually occurs within a matter of minutes after contact with the insect venom. The reaction can result in death if the necessary medication that reverses the reaction is not immediately available. See *Anaphylaxis,* Chapter 4.

Symptoms of a *severe allergic reaction* include:

- Flushed skin
- Hives with welts
- Sudden sense of uneasiness and anxiety

Avoiding Insect Stings

There are ways for children and staff to reduce the chance of being stung while outdoors. These are especially important for the allergic child.

- A nonallergic adult should destroy any nests that appear around the building. Check under eaves and windowsills.
- Check for nests in other locations where children play, such as old tree stumps, auto tires that are part of a playground, holes in the ground, and around rotting wood.
- Allergic children should not play outside alone during the months when stinging insects are active.
- Sneakers are safer than sandals for allergic children.
- Clothing for allergic children should not have bright floral prints. Colors such as white or khaki are best. Avoid loose-fitting clothes because they can trap a stinging insect.
- Avoid perfumes, hairsprays, or other products with scents that might make the child attractive to insects.
- When eating outdoors, be aware that stinging insects are attracted to foods and can enter soft drink cans. These foods especially attract insects: tuna, peanut butter and jelly sandwiches, watermelon, and melting ice cream.
- Avoid garbage cans and dumpsters because they attract insects.
- If an insect is near you, do not swat or run since such actions can trigger an attack. Walk away slowly. If you have disturbed a nest and the insects swarm around you, lie face down and cover your head with your arms. Teach this technique to children.
- A severe allergic reaction to an insect sting is immediate and life-threatening. Therefore, an allergic child's emergency kit should be kept close at hand when the child is playing outdoors during insect season. An allergic child should also wear a medical alert necklace or bracelet to alert a rescuer who might find the child unresponsive.

- Dizziness
- Swelling, sometimes severe, at the sting site and elsewhere, especially face, lips, or tongue
- Abdominal or stomach cramps and diarrhea

- Tightness in the chest
- Wheezing or difficulty breathing caused by swelling in the throat that can progress to a complete blockage of the airway
- Bluish or grayish skin color around lips and mouth
- Loss of consciousness

What to Do

1. Examine the sting site for a stinger left in the skin. Only honey bees leave the stinger with the venom sac attached. It must be removed, because it continues to inject venom for 2 or 3 minutes longer if left in the skin. Scrape it away from the site with a fingernail, nail file, table knife blade, or similar object. Avoid removing the stinger sac with fingers or tweezers, because this squeezes the sac and injects more venom.

2. Apply a baking soda and water paste to the site to reduce the stinging pain. Baking soda neutralizes acidic venom. If you know the stinging insect was a wasp, put vinegar or lemon juice on the sting site to neutralize that alkaline venom. Later, apply calamine lotion to help control itching.

3. Apply ice or a cold pack wrapped in a wet cloth (to protect the skin) for 15 to 20 minutes. This slows the absorption of venom and relieves pain.

4. Observe the child for signs of an allergic reaction. A delayed reaction can occur up to 24 hours after the sting. For a mild reaction, call the child's parent immediately. If a severe allergic reaction, or anaphylaxis, occurs:

   - Send someone to call for emergency medical help. Emergency medical technicians carry an allergic emergency kit in their rescue vehicles.
   - Use an allergic child's allergic emergency kit if you have it on hand and have been instructed in how to use it. At least one staff member in the center should be taught to use the kit. It should be stored with first aid supplies in the child care center at room temperature. This is not a routine item in all first aid kits, but rather a prescription drug intended specifically for the allergic child who is having a severe allergic reaction. Older children should have their kit with them at all times. The kit contains an easy-

to-use mechanism that administers the correct dose of the drug. A second dose of medication might be necessary while waiting for emergency medical help to arrive.

- Check and monitor the ABCDs and treat accordingly. Swelling in the throat makes rescue breathing difficult.
- Position an unresponsive child on the left side in the recovery position. Position a conscious child who is having difficulty breathing in a sitting position to make breathing easier.
- Position the sting site so that it is lower than the level of the heart.
- Notify the child's parent.

The Soft Drink Can Sting

Children who are playing outdoors and walk away from their soft drink or juice cans might receive an unpleasant surprise when they come back for another sip. In a number of instances, a stinging insect attracted to the sweetness has landed on the soda can lid, fallen into the beverage, and ended up in the child's mouth, delivering a sting to the mouth or throat. A sting in this location can cause throat swelling even in a nonallergic child.

As an ounce of prevention, pour beverages into plastic cups when outdoors. This way, you and the child can see that no insects are in the beverage.

Should a sting occur inside the mouth, give the child plenty of ice chips to suck on for pain relief. Avoid ice cubes in young children because they are slippery and can block the airway if they slip to the back of the throat. If you know it is a bee sting, have the child hold in the mouth a baking soda and water mixture of 1 teaspoon baking soda to 8 ounces of water. Repeatedly hold in the mouth and rinse for several minutes to help neutralize the acidic venom.

Snakebite

Snakes are shy creatures that avoid humans and tend only to bite when surprised or cornered. Although interesting to some children, most children prefer to stay away from snakes and should be taught to be cautious around them. Snakes are wild animals, and their behavior is unpredictable.

Both poisonous and nonpoisonous snakes bite people. Most snakebites occur on the upper extremities and happen when people approach the snake, whether to try to capture, relocate, play with, or even kill it. Of approximately 7,000 bites from poisonous snakes each year, only about a dozen result in death. The highest incidence of snakebite occurs in children and teenagers. Children experience more severe reactions to poisonous snakebites than do teens or adults.

Only four species of snakes in the United States are poisonous: rattlesnake, copperhead, water moccasin, and coral snake. Rattlesnakes are responsible for over two thirds of venomous snake bites and almost all of the deaths. The most important part of treating a poisonous snakebite is getting the antivenin into the child as soon as possible after the bite.

Pit Viper Snakebite

Rattlesnakes, copperheads, and water moccasins are known as pit vipers. They share three common characteristics:

- A triangle-shaped, flat head that is wider than the neck
- Slit-like eyes
- Heat-sensitive "pit" located between each eye and nostril

Keep Kids and Snakes Apart

Poisonous snakes exist in all parts of the United States but are the biggest problem in areas where there are large numbers of them.

- Be aware of the poisonous species in your area, and avoid taking young children to locations near woods, grasses, or desert where snakes live.
- Teach children not to poke into crevices or holes, under rocks, or around logs.
- Do not allow children to tease or poke at a snake, even a dead one.
- If you come upon a snake you believe to be poisonous, immediately retrace your steps in the opposite direction or make a very large circle to go around it.
- Let a snake know you are coming by making noise as you walk along.

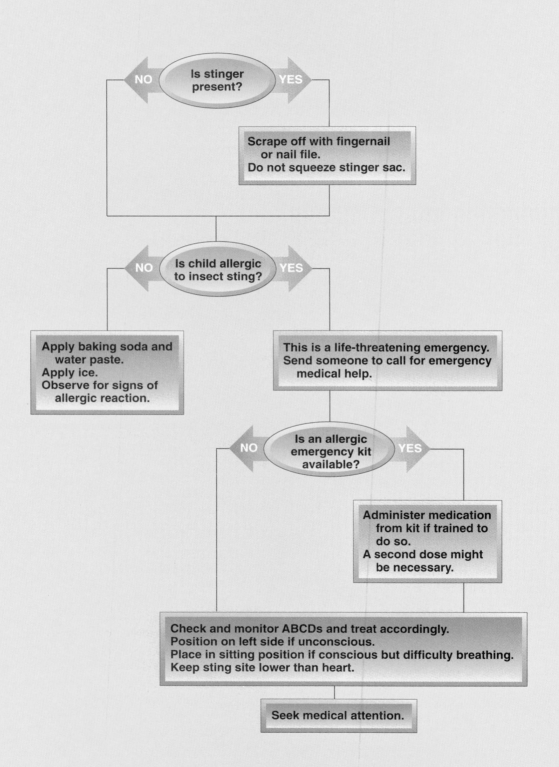

Is stinger present?

NO

YES

Scrape off with fingernail
or nail file.
Do not squeeze stinger sac.

Is child allergic
to insect sting?

NO

YES

Apply baking soda and
water paste.
Apply ice.
Observe for signs of
allergic reaction.

This is a life-threatening emergency.
Send someone to call for emergency
medical help.

Is an allergic
emergency kit
available?

NO

YES

Administer medication
from kit if trained to
do so.
A second dose might
be necessary.

Check and monitor ABCDs and treat accordingly.
Position on left side if unconscious.
Place in sitting position if conscious but difficulty breathing.
Keep sting site lower than heart.

Seek medical attention.

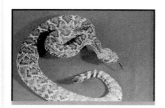

Rattlesnake

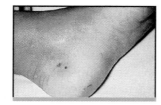

Rattlesnake bite showing the two-prong fang marks

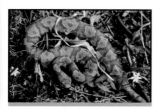

Copperhead snake

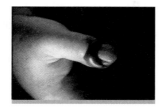

Copperhead bite after 2 hours

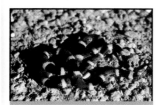

Coral snake

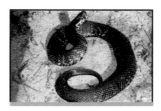

Cottonmouth water moccasin snake

Their venom affects the circulatory system and causes destruction of the local tissue around the bite. The same antivenin is administered for all three pit viper bites.

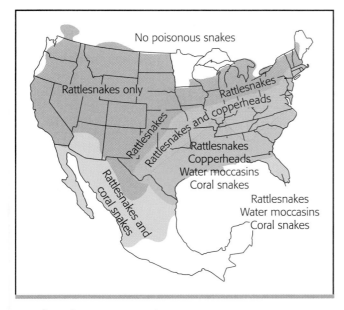

Location of venomous snakes

What to Look For

- Severe burning pain at the bite site
- Distinctive bite markings of two puncture wounds from the fangs and two sets of teeth marks extending back from the fang marks
- Swelling that starts quickly and may eventually involve the entire arm or leg
- Discoloration and blood-filled blisters develop several hours after the bite
- In severe cases: nausea, vomiting, weakness, blurred vision, breathing difficulties, seizures, and shock
- For one in five bites, no venom is injected from the fangs. This is called a dry bite and is a much less serious injury.

What to Do

1. Get the child away from the snake. Children, in particular, can be immobilized by fright and risk being bitten again. Even some dead snakes have a bite reaction for up to 30 minutes. If possible, try to identify whether the snake is a pit viper or a coral snake, because of the difference in their antivenins.
2. Send someone to call for emergency medical help. The child's most *urgent* need is to receive antivenin. You can also call your local poison control center as a resource. Especially in parts of the country where poisonous snakes are populous, poison control centers are very knowledgeable about poisonous snakebites.
3. Keep the child calm. If the child must be moved, carry the child rather than allow walking. Have the child lie down, position the arm below the level of the heart, and remain still, which helps to slow the absorption of the venom into the bloodstream.
4. Gently wash the bite with soap and water.
5. Notify the child's parent.

DO NOT

- attempt to cut the skin and suck the venom, because you might cut too deeply, your mouth bacteria can infect the wound, and you might inadvertently swallow the venom.
- apply a constriction band or a tourniquet above the snakebite site.

Signs and Symptoms of Infection

Some bites leave wounds that can become infected. Check the wound regularly and contact the child's parent if you note any of the following signs and symptoms. The child's health care provider should then be contacted.

- Throbbing pain
- Swelling
- Skin around the wound is warm to the touch
- Redness around the wound
- Red streaks leading away from the wound
- Enlarged lymph nodes
- Pus
- Fever

Coral Snakebite

The coral snake is the most venomous snake in the United States but rarely bites people. It is characterized by:

- A colorful body with a series of bright red, yellow, and black bands. Every other band is yellow.
- A black snout and round eyes

The coral snake is smaller than any of the three pit vipers and has short fangs. It tends to bite and hang on to its victim with a chewing motion rather than to bite and let go in the way that a pit viper does. Its venom causes a generalized reaction affecting the nervous system. First aid for a coral snakebite is similar to that of any poisonous snakebite; however, bites from the coral snake are treated with a different antivenin than those from pit vipers.

What to Look For

- Most signs and symptoms are not at the bite site and do not appear for 1 to 4 hours after the bite.
- The bite is usually located on a small finger or toe or in the webbing between the fingers because the coral snake has a tiny mouth and teeth.
- Slight pain and swelling at the site of the bite
- Drowsiness, tremors, and heavy drooling develop after the first few hours.
- After a few more hours, blurred vision, drooping eyelids, slurred speech, seizures (in younger children), and difficulty breathing begin.

Nonpoisonous Snakes

Nonpoisonous snakes' tooth markings are horseshoe-shaped on the skin. Some nonpoisonous snakes do inject venom, but it causes only a local reaction. However, if you are unsure of a snake species, especially in an area heavily populated by poisonous snakes, assume it is poisonous and make arrangements to have the child taken to an emergency medical facility where a health care provider can make a determination by the fang markings on the child's skin. You can also call your local poison control center as a resource. Especially in parts of the country where poisonous snakes are populous, poison control centers are very knowledgeable about snakebites.

Treat a nonpoisonous snakebite as a puncture wound. Wash with soap and water and encourage a small amount of bleeding by gently squeezing the area while washing. Contact the child's parent and health care provider. Observe the healing wound daily for signs of infection.

Spider Bites

Watching a spider descend on its silk or spin its web is a fascinating activity for adults and children alike. Children should be taught to enjoy watching spiders but to be cautious of them, because a few are poisonous to humans. Nearly all spiders are venomous: this is how they kill the insects they eat. Those that have fangs long enough to bite humans include the black widow, brown recluse, and tarantula spiders. Death from a spider bite is rare in North America, but recovery from a bite can be prolonged for children. Spiders prefer places that are dark, such as the basement, a barn, a wood pile, or the undersides of rocks. A spider bite may be a painful surprise or may go unnoticed until signs and symptoms begin to develop.

Black Widow Spider

Black widow spiders are found worldwide. Only the female black widow bites. She is jet black and has a red spot, often in the shape of an hourglass, on the underside of the abdomen. The only spider bite for which there is antivenin is the black widow's. Children should always receive this antivenin, because the bite is especially toxic to them and several bites can cause death.

What to Look For

- A sharp local pain initially when the spider bites followed by a dull, numbing pain. Some children are not aware of being bitten.

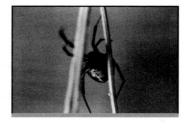

Black widow spider

- Two small red spots are the fang marks.
- Several hours of severe abdominal pain caused by muscle spasms when the bite is in the lower part of the body or legs, or severe pain in the shoulders, back, or chest when the bite is on the upper body or arms.
- Nausea and vomiting
- Fever and profuse sweating
- Headache and dizziness
- Breathing difficulties caused by paralysis of the breathing muscles can develop up to 24 hours after the bite.

Brown Recluse Spider

The brown recluse spider is tan or brown with a brown or purplish fiddle-shaped mark on its back. The bite is especially toxic to young children. It causes extensive damage around the bite, which is extremely painful. It heals slowly over 1 to 2 months and needs to be watched closely for signs of infection. There is no antivenin for this bite.

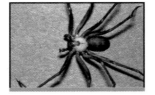

Brown recluse spider

What to Look For

The actual bite might go unnoticed or produce only mild pain.

- Within 6 to 8 hours, tenderness, inflammation and pain develop and a blister appears. Tissue damage in the blister area will become severe.
- Within 12 to 24 hours, flu-like symptoms develop, with high fever, chills, cramps, joint pain, nausea, and vomiting.
- After 48 hours, the blister begins to turn white as the tissue destruction intensifies and

worsens for about 1 week. Pain can be intolerable.

Tarantula

These are large, hairy, and scary-looking spiders that children run from if they see them. The bite is painful when it occurs, but it causes only local tissue damage. There is no systemic reaction throughout the body. Children are much more susceptible to the toxin than are adults. There is no antivenin for the tarantula bite.

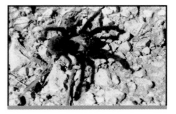

Tarantula

What to Do for Spider Bites

1. Identify or capture the spider, if possible. It is okay if the body is crushed. Some bites go unnoticed for hours, making identification unlikely.
2. Wash the bite with soap and water.
3. Place ice or a cold pack wrapped in a wet cloth over the bite to relieve pain.
4. Have the child examined in an emergency medical facility immediately or, in some cases, as soon as the signs and symptoms become apparent.
5. Notify the child's parent.

DO NOT

- apply a constricting band to a spider bite. In all cases but the black widow bite, the venom does not affect tissue beyond the site of the bite. Black widow venom, which can cause a reaction in other parts of the body, acts so swiftly that applying a constricting band is ineffective.

Scorpion Stings

Most children fear scorpions because of their ugly appearance and reputation for a menacing sting. Scorpions look like tiny lobsters with a poisonous stinger in the tail that arches up over the back. In the southwestern United States where scorpions are common, their stings kill more children than do snakebites. Antivenin is available in emergency medical facilities only in the state of Arizona where the scorpion population is quite large.

What to Look For

- Immediate pain and burning around the sting site, followed by pain, numbness, and tingling spreading up the extremity

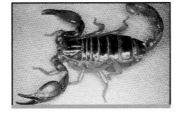

Scorpion

- Within an hour: headache, high fever, nausea, dizziness, and increased salivation
- Shock in severe cases
- Severe cases usually appear only in young children and may advance to include seizures, paralysis or spasms of affected muscles and jaw muscles, excessive salivation, facial twitching, difficulty with speech and vision, and breathing difficulties.
- The first 3 hours after the sting are the most critical hours in terms of severity of reaction and survival.
- Symptoms can last up to 24 hours.

What to Do

1. Send someone to call for emergency medical help.
2. Monitor the ABCDs and treat accordingly.
3. Wash the site with soap and water.
4. Apply a cold pack or ice wrapped in a cloth.

Tick Bites

Most tick bites are harmless, although ticks occasionally carry diseases, such as Rocky Mountain spotted fever and Lyme disease. Ticks attach themselves to clothing or the exposed skin of a person walking in the woods or tall grasses. A tick bite is often not felt. If unnoticed, the tick can remain attached and embedded for days.

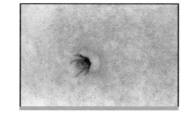

Embedded tick

Diseases are transmitted after the tick bites the skin and while it is feeding. As ticks draw blood for food, some can increase their size by 10 times or more. Checking children and pets regularly for ticks and removing a tick promptly are

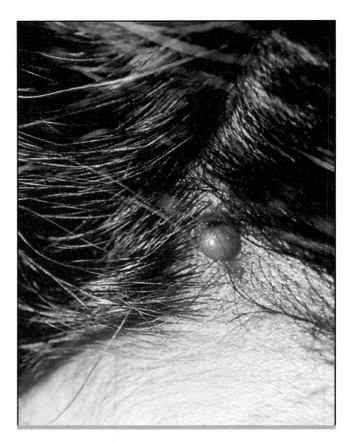

An engorged tick at the hair line

two important steps in preventing both a tick bite and any of the illnesses that they can transmit. Remove a tick using the following method:

What to Do

1. Use tweezers rather than fingertips. Grasp the tick close to the skin surface where the mouth parts are attached. Pull gently and firmly until the tick lets go. Do not twist or jerk, because this might leave part of the tick in the skin.
2. Wash the area with soap and water. Dab rubbing alcohol on the bite area.
3. Apply ice or a cold pack wrapped in a wet cloth (to protect the skin).
4. Apply calamine lotion for itching.

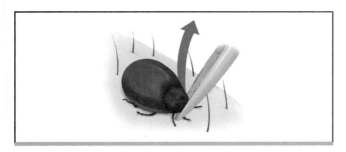

Remove a tick with tweezers.

5. Notify the child's parent at the end of the day.
6. Both child care providers and parents should observe the bite site for a doughnut-shaped or other rash or signs of infection for the next several weeks. Also observe the child for flu-like symptoms, such as fever, muscle aches, or joint pain and for sensitivity to bright light. The child's health care provider should be contacted about any symptoms that develop for up to 4 weeks after a tick bite.

DO NOT

- attempt to remove a tick by coating it with petroleum jelly or fingernail polish, soaking it in alcohol, or holding a hot match against it. These methods are likely to be ineffective and some are not safe.

Tick Bite Prevention

- Cover legs with long pants tucked into socks, tuck in long-sleeved shirts at the waist, and wear sneakers instead of sandals when walking in tall grass, woods, or fields. Ticks are most easily spotted on light-colored clothing.
- Stay on trails whenever possible.

- Check children's skin daily for ticks if they play in these areas. Pay special attention to the folds of the skin and the scalp and the back of the neck. Removing the tick within the first 24 hours greatly reduces the risk of infection.
- Contact your local health department to find out if deer ticks are prevalent in your area.
- Check pets for ticks. They can carry ticks and are also susceptible to disease. Use tick control products recommended by your veterinarian.

Continued next page

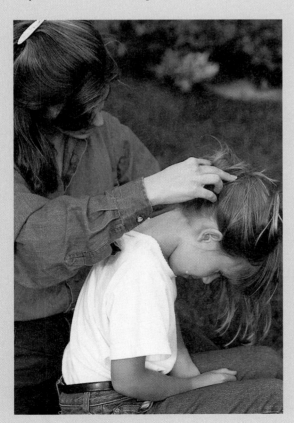

Checking for ticks

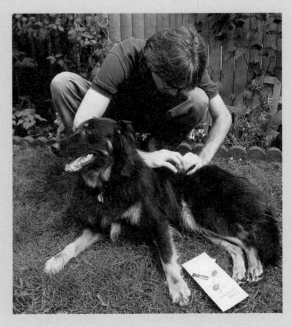

Check pets for ticks, too.

Tick Bite Prevention, Continued

- Parents may use over-the-counter insect repellents that contain no more than 10% DEET on infants and small children. DEET on the skin irritates ticks and causes them to drop off. A repellent containing 0.5% Permethrin, a pesticide, should be applied to the clothing only, never to the skin. Child care providers should not expose children in their care to situations where the use of DEET would be necessary.

- Spray insect repellents only when outdoors, use sparingly, and wash hands after applying. Never apply it to the face, to an open wound or cut, or to the hands or arms of a child who is likely to put them in the mouth.

Lyme Disease

Disease from an infected tick is not a new problem. Lyme disease is a relatively new name for a disease that was first identified early in the 20th century. It has received a great deal of publicity in recent years in an attempt to alert the public to its symptoms and to help diagnose the illness in its early stage, when it is easily treated. Lyme disease is a bacterial infection transmitted by the bite of an infected deer tick or western blacklegged tick. In some areas of the United States, this tick is also known as a bear tick or sheep tick. The deer tick is smaller than the more common dog or wood tick. It can be as small as the head of a pin and when engorged with blood is somewhat larger.

Lyme disease has been found in nearly all of the United States, although it tends to concentrate in the Northeast, northern Midwest, Pacific Northwest, and California. The incidence in the Southeast is on the rise. The range of the disease is expanding as the ticks are carried farther inland by animals and birds.

Ticks carrying Lyme disease are not found on sandy beaches.

Humans can contract the disease when they are out in the fields and woods where the deer tick lives. The months of greatest risk are May through August. During these months the infected ticks are in their nymph, or infancy, stage and are so tiny (about the size of a period on this page) that they easily go undetected. In warmer regions of the United States, the risk of Lyme disease can exist year-round. The Centers for Disease Control reports that in a recent year, 9,677 cases were reported to state health departments nationwide. More than 1,000 of those cases occurred in children under age 10. Children between ages 5 and 9 are the most vulnerable, because they are likely to play in wooded or grassy areas in warmer weather without a parent with them to ensure that proper tick precautions are taken.

As with other ticks, the deer tick attaches itself to the clothing or exposed skin of a child walking in

Continued next page

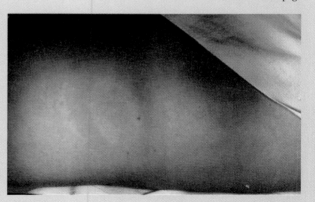

Unengorged and engorged deer ticks (seven times actual size)

Lyme disease rash

the fields or woods where the deer tick lives. The Lyme disease bacteria is transmitted to the child after the tick bites, while it is becoming engorged as it draws blood for food. It is believed that the tick must be attached to the body for at least 24 hours for the infection to be transmitted. Only a small number of deer ticks are actually infected with the Lyme disease bacterium. It is important for people to realize that although the danger of Lyme disease is very real, the risk of contracting it is actually very small.

Early signs and symptoms of Lyme disease can appear from 1 to 4 weeks after the deer tick bite. Treatment at this stage is very effective and the disease lasts for about 2 weeks.

- In approximately 60% to 75% of Lyme disease cases, a red rash develops at the site of the bite. This important early finding helps to diagnose the disease promptly. The rash usually appears first as a large circle and then begins to resembles a bull's eye or a doughnut as the red color of the center begins to fade leaving an outer circle of redness. If left untreated, the rash disappears in several weeks.

- Additional early symptoms of Lyme disease, which can be mistaken for a flu-like illness, are: headache, fatigue, fever, chills, swollen glands, stiff neck, and aching muscles or joints.

If not caught early, signs and symptoms disappear and reappear weeks or months later. These later signs and symptoms of Lyme disease are more serious. Recovery from this stage of the disease occurs more slowly, but children recover more quickly than adults.

- Painful swelling of joints, often the knees
- Heart problems causing an irregular heartbeat, dizziness, and weakness
- Nervous system problems causing headache, neck stiffness, difficulty concentrating, and poor coordination

A Lyme disease diagnosis is usually based on symptoms that the child and parents report. A blood test can help to confirm it but is not always reliable. Lyme disease is treated with antibiotics.

Name _____ Course _____ Date _____

1. Circle true (T) or false (F) for each of the following statements about bites.

   T   F   a. An animal bite that does not break the skin can become infected.

   T   F   b. Both warm-blooded and cold-blooded animals can be infected with rabies.

   T   F   c. Family pets are the leading rabies carriers.

   T   F   d. The rabies virus is passed through the saliva of an infected animal.

   T   F   e. A small amount of bleeding while washing a wound helps to clean it.

   T   F   f. A spayed or neutered dog is more likely to bite than an unneutered dog.

   T   F   g. Raccoons are responsible for almost all animal bites in the United States.

2. List three signs or symptoms of infection in a bite wound.

   a. _____
   b. _____
   c. _____

3. A baby raccoon wanders out of the woods and approaches children playing in the sandbox in the play yard. They think the animal is cute and want to pet it. What should you be concerned about?

   _____

4. Why might you think that there is something wrong with the animal?

   _____

5. A child in your home care program runs into the yard next door to retrieve a ball, surprising a leashed dog, and is bitten. The bite is not deep, but it does break the skin. List three first aid steps you would take:

   a. _____
   b. _____
   c. _____

6. Which of the following animals are most likely to carry rabies? Circle yes (Y) or no (N).

   Y   N   a. Skunk
   Y   N   b. Turtle
   Y   N   c. Raccoon
   Y   N   d. Bat
   Y   N   e. Wasp
   Y   N   f. Guinea pig
   Y   N   g. Immunized dog
   Y   N   h. Snake
   Y   N   i. Fox
   Y   N   j. Spider

7. Five-year-old Carlos is stung by a bee. He runs to you crying and holding his hand. Your first aid includes which of the following? Circle yes (Y) or no (N).

   Y   N   a. Remove the stinger with tweezers or fingers.

   Y   N   b. Wash the sting site with soap and water.

   Y   N   c. Place a warm pack over the sting site.

   Y   N   d. Observe for signs and symptoms of an allergic reaction.

8. Why is it important to remove the stinger?

   _____
   _____

9. What can you do to help relieve pain after a bee sting?

   _____ and _____

10. List three signs or symptoms of a normal skin reaction to an insect sting.

    a. _____
    b. _____
    c. _____

11. A boy with a known allergy to bees is stung while your group of children is coming inside from the play yard. He is crying and holding his leg. Within minutes you notice hives on his chest and welts forming on his neck. He complains that he is having difficulty swallowing. What care is important to provide during this emergency?

    a. _____

    b. _____

    c. _____

    d. _____

12. Circle true (T) or false (F) for each statement about snakebites.

    T   F   a. Elevate a snake bite wound above the level of the heart to reduce absorption of the venom.

    T   F   b. It is possible to be bitten by a dead snake.

    T   F   c. If you are unsure of a snake's species, assume it is poisonous.

    T   F   d. A distinguishing characteristic of a poisonous snakebite is that there are two puncture wounds at the bite site.

    T   F   e. The child's most urgent need after a poisonous snakebite is to receive a tetanus shot.

    T   F   f. The same antivenin is used for all poisonous snakebites.

13. The only poisonous spider bite for which antivenin is available is

    _____.

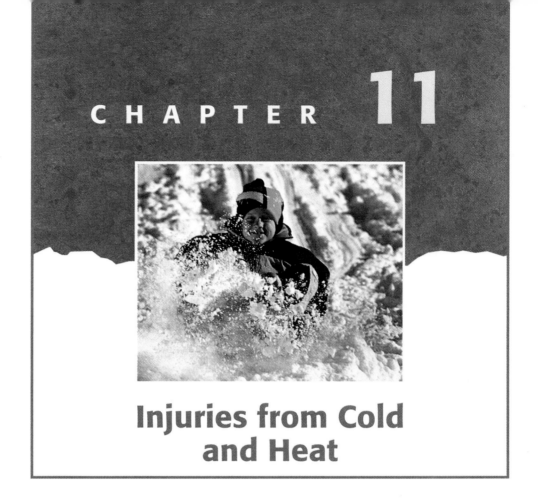

CHAPTER 11

Injuries from Cold and Heat

Injury and illness caused by excesses in outside temperature can create problems for children.

Cold-Related Injuries

Outdoor play is a healthy activity enjoyed by most young children and should be encouraged even during the colder weather months. However, some winter weather conditions can sneak up on a lost child or a child busily intent on play and have dangerous consequences to health.

Frostbite

Frostbite occurs when skin and underlying tissues are damaged by exposure to temperatures below freezing. The tissue freezes and the blood supply slows so much that there is too little oxygen getting to the tissue. Both air temperature and length of exposure determine the extent of the damage.

Children are more susceptible to frostbite than adults, because they have less body fat to insulate them. Frostbite is often seen on hands, cheeks, ears, noses, and feet. In severe cases, tissue dies and must be amputated.

Frostbite is an uncommon occurrence in a child care center or a home care setting, because the exposure conditions necessary for this extent of damage are rarely, if ever, experienced in a well-supervised situation. However, the threat of the serious damage of frostbite serves as a reminder of just how important it is to monitor children outdoors in cold weather both

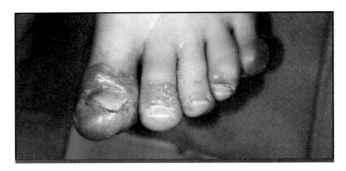

Blistered, frostbitten toes

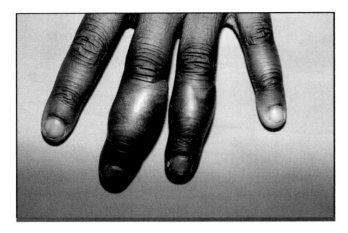

Frostbitten fingers, 6 hours after rewarming in 108°F water

for length of exposure and for keeping mittens and hats on.

What to Look For

Initially, exposed or underprotected skin feels cold and mildly painful to the child who is outdoors and focused on play or other activity. The pain subsides as the skin becomes numb, if exposure continues. The signs and symptoms of mild frostbite are most apparent when the child comes indoors.

Mild Frostbite
- Coldness and numbness of the affected area
- Tingling and burning of the affected area
- Aching or throbbing pain
- Milky-white or grayish-yellow skin color
- Waxy-looking skin
- Skin feels hard, but tissue underneath feels soft
- No blisters

Severe Frostbite
- Swelling of the frostbitten area as it starts to thaw
- Skin color pale blue, red, purple, or blue-black after thawing begins
- Blistered skin
- Stiffness or difficulty moving the body part
- Severe aching and throbbing pain
- Skin and underlying tissue feel solid and hard

What to Do

1. Bring the child indoors and remove clothing and jewelry from the affected area.
2. Handle the area very gently while you examine it for frostbite.
3. Leave intact blisters alone, and cover blisters that rupture with a sterile gauze pad.

DO NOT
- **break blisters on frostbitten skin.**

4. Slightly elevate the area to decrease pain and swelling. Place gauze between the fingers or toes to prevent them from sticking together and to absorb moisture.
5. Have the child taken to an emergency medical facility immediately.

Preventing Frostbite and Frostnip

Frostbite and frostnip occur when children are playing outdoors or enjoying winter sports for long periods of time and are inadequately dressed for the cold and fail to notice their developing symptoms. Take the following precautions to prevent either of these conditions from occurring:

- Dress appropriately. See *Dressing for Winter.*
- Observe for white spots forming on cheeks that might indicate mild frostbite.
- Bring a child indoors immediately if complaining of a cold, numb, tingling, or painful area on the body.
- Check the temperature and limit outdoor play time accordingly during the cold-weather months. See *How Cold Is It?*
- Teach children about the importance of frostbite prevention because, once frostbitten, the injured body part is more susceptible to future episodes of frostbite and continues to be extremely sensitive to cold . The child can experience tingling, loss of feeling, and pain during cold weather for many years.

FROSTBITE AND FROSTNIP

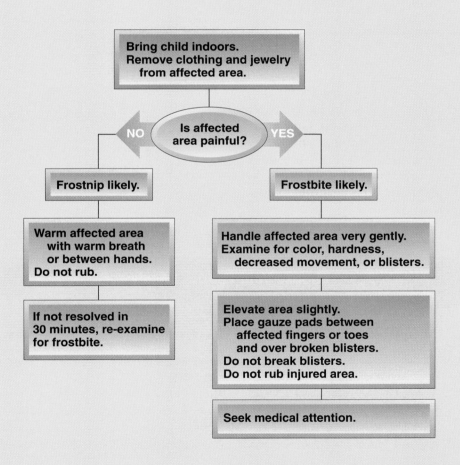

Bring child indoors.
Remove clothing and jewelry
from affected area.

NO — Is affected
area painful? — **YES**

Frostnip likely.

Frostbite likely.

Warm affected area
with warm breath
or between hands.
Do not rub.

Handle affected area very gently.
Examine for color, hardness,
decreased movement, or blisters.

If not resolved in
30 minutes, re-examine
for frostbite.

Elevate area slightly.
Place gauze pads between
affected fingers or toes
and over broken blisters.
Do not break blisters.
Do not rub injured area.

Seek medical attention.

DO NOT

- attempt to rewarm the area yourself by using warm water, a heating pad, a blow dryer, heat from a fireplace, hands in underarms, or other poorly measurable heat sources. Leave this care to medical professionals, who will warm the area rapidly using a carefully controlled technique.
- rub the area in an attempt to stimulate circulation. This could result in further damage to fragile skin and in ice crystals causing rupture of underlying tissue.
- rub snow on the area.
- allow a child to walk on feet that might be frostbitten.

Frostnip

Frostnip is caused by exposure to the cold but is less serious than frostbite, because the damage does not penetrate as deeply. It occurs on the same areas as frostbite—hands, cheeks, ears, noses, and feet. However, of the two cold-related injuries, it is more likely that a child will experience frostnip than frostbite, because frostnip requires a shorter exposure time to develop.

Dressing for Winter

Dress children carefully for winter outdoor activities, so they will be untouched by cold weather-related injuries. Child care providers should notify parents of the cold-weather clothing that they would like to see the children come dressed in to school every day. Parents should dress their child as is appropriate for their climate. Make certain that children in your care:

- Wear boots when playing in the snow to prevent frostbite to toes. Water-repellent boots with a thermal interior are the warmest and driest.
- Wear snow pants, because the insulation they provide keeps pants dry and legs warm.
- Wear mittens rather than gloves, because mittens keep fingers together, keeping them warmer.
- Keep their hats on their heads, because a large percentage of body heat loss occurs through the head.
- Apply petroleum jelly to exposed areas of the face to prevent chapping.

Choose Your Fabrics Wisely

	Advantages	Disadvantages	Wear As
Wool	Stretches without damage; insulates well even when wet	Heavy weight; absorbs moisture; may irritate skin	Layer 1, 2, or 3
Cotton	Comfortable and lightweight	Absorbs moisture	Layer 1 or 2
Silk	Extremely lightweight and durable; very good insulator; washes well	More expensive; does not transfer moisture quickly	Layer 1
Polypropylene	Lightweight; transfers moisture quickly and dries quickly	Does not insulate well; surface may pill	Layer 1 or 2
Down	Durable, lightweight; most effective insulator by weight	Expensive; loses insulating quality when wet; difficult to dry	Layer 2 or 3 (especially in dry, extreme cold)
Nylon	Lightweight; wind- and water-resistant; durable	May not allow perspiration to evaporate	Layer 3
Synthetic Polyester Insulation	Does not absorb moisture, therefore insulates even when wet	Heavier than down; does not compress as well	Layer 2 or 3 (especially in wet weather)

Adapted from *National Safety Council*, Family Safety & Health.

Frostnip is characterized by redness, discomfort, and a tingling awareness that the body part feels uncomfortably cold. You might also notice a white patch on the cheek or nose. If ignored, frostnip can develop into frostbite.

What to Do

If you suspect frostnip, cover the area and have the child come indoors immediately. Warm hands and fingers by holding them in your hands, blowing warm breath on them, or having the child hold them in the child's underarms. The skin may continue to appear red and feel tingly for a while after rewarming, but it should not be painful. Do not rub a frostnipped area. If the child complains of pain, especially 30 minutes or more after treatment, re-examine the area for signs of frostbite.

Hypothermia

Hypothermia is a dangerous condition in which the body loses more heat than it can produce, causing the core body temperature to drop below 95°F. It is caused by prolonged exposure to cold air or cold water. Hypothermia slows the activity of all tissues of the body, and if the exposure is lengthy or the body temperature drops too low, the child might not recover. Children are especially susceptible to

hypothermia, because they have less fat than adults and small muscles, which do not create as successful a shivering response. Infants do not shiver at all.

A child who becomes hypothermic is outdoors for a very long time and/or is inadequately prepared for the weather conditions. A child can fall through ice or become separated from adults on a walk and spend several hours outdoors before being rescued. In these conditions, hypothermia can be accompanied by frostbite.

But even in summer, hypothermia dangers exist for swimmers who remain in the water too long and for those caught underdressed by wet and windy weather or in a wet sleeping bag. Wet conditions, whether from rain, snow, or perspiration, increase heat loss from the body and thus are often associated with hypothermia. A 50°F temperature in wet conditions is more dangerous than a 20°F temperature in dry conditions. Wind also increases heat loss, so pay attention to the wind-chill factor when making outdoor plans in winter.

What to Look For

Early symptoms (with core body temperature of 90°F or above)

- Shivering (the body's way of increasing its temperature)
- Feeling very cold, especially in the abdomen and back
- Confusion
- Clumsiness and lack of coordination
- Slurred speech
- Slow pulse

Later symptoms (with core body temperature below 90°F)

- Shivering stops
- Skin very cold and appears blue or gray
- Muscles become rigid
- Irrational behavior and speech
- Decreased pulse and breathing
- Dilated pupils
- Unconsciousness and coma

What to Do

1. Send someone to call for emergency medical help. This is a true emergency and the child

How Cold Is It?

Wind can make the temperature feel lower than the thermometer registers. If the thermometer reads 20°F and the wind speed is 20 mph, the exposure is comparable to −10°F. This is called the wind-chill factor. A rough measure of wind speed is: If you feel the wind on your face, the speed is about 10 mph; if small branches move or dust or snow is raised, 20 mph; if large branches are moving, 30 mph; and if a whole tree bends, about 40 mph.

Determine the wind-chill factor by:

1. Estimating the wind speed by checking for the signs described above.
2. Looking at a thermometer reading outdoors.
3. Matching the estimated wind speed with the thermometer reading in the "Wind-Chill Factor" table.

Wind-Chill Factor

Estimated Wind Speed (in mph)	Actual Thermometer Reading (°F)											
	50	40	30	20	10	0	−10	−20	−30	−40	−50	−60
	Equivalent Temperature (°F)											
Calm	50	40	30	20	10	0	−10	−20	−30	−40	−50	−60
5	40	37	27	16	6	−5	−15	−26	−36	−47	−57	−68
10	40	28	16	4	−9	−24	−33	−46	−58	−70	−83	−95
15	36	22	9	−5	−18	−32	−45	−58	−72	−85	−99	−112
20	32	18	4	−10	−25	−39	−53	−67	−82	−96	−110	−124
25	30	16	0	−15	−29	−44	−59	−74	−88	−104	−118	−133
30	25	13	−2	−18	−33	−48	−63	−79	−94	−109	−125	−140
35	27	11	−4	−20	−35	−51	−67	−82	−98	−113	−129	−145
40*	26	10	−6	−21	−37	−53	−69	−85	−100	−116	−132	−148

Little danger (for properly clothed person). Maximum danger of false sense of security. → Increasing danger. (Flesh may freeze within 1 minute.) → Great danger. (Flesh may freeze within 30 seconds.) →

*Wind speeds greater than 40 mph have little additional effect.

must be treated in an emergency medical facility immediately.

2. If unresponsive, check and monitor the ABCDs and treat accordingly. You will need to take extra time (30 seconds or more) checking for the pulse, because it is slow and difficult to detect.

3. If emergency medical help will arrive promptly, leave the child in the location found. Prevent further heat loss by insulating the child from the ground, using jackets, blankets, or newspapers. Cover the child with a blanket and allow the child to shiver.

4. If emergency medical help will not arrive promptly, move the child indoors. Handle the child gently and as little as possible because rough handling can cause the heart to stop. Cover the child with a blanket and allow the child to shiver.

5. Keep the child lying flat.

6. Change the child into dry clothes if clothes are wet.

7. Put a hat on the child even if indoors. Nearly half of the body's heat loss is through the head.

Leave rewarming to the medical professionals, who can minimize the rewarming risks to the heart. Tra-

ditional methods of warming a child, such as skin-to-skin contact and using a heating pad, are not only ineffective but can be dangerous, because these methods stop the shivering process by warming the skin surface without warming the vital internal organs. Shivering helps the body rewarm itself from the inside out by causing muscles to contract. This is the body's natural response to a drop in body temperature. Chances of survival are good if the child is conscious when found.

DO NOT

- massage the child's arms or legs or handle the body roughly, because it can cause the heart to stop.
- elevate the legs, because cold blood from the legs will flow into the core of the body.
- allow the child to walk.
- give anything to eat or drink. Warm drinks cause skin capillaries to dilate and heat to be lost.
- use skin-to-skin rewarming or a heating pad. This warms the skin but inhibits shivering.

HYPOTHERMIA

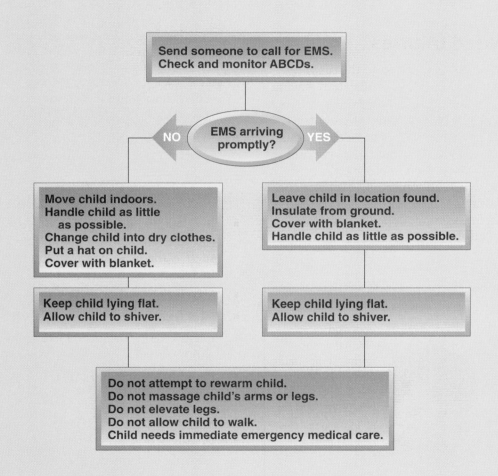

Send someone to call for EMS.
Check and monitor ABCDs.

EMS arriving promptly?

NO

YES

NO branch:
Move child indoors.
Handle child as little
  as possible.
Change child into dry clothes.
Put a hat on child.
Cover with blanket.

Keep child lying flat.
Allow child to shiver.

YES branch:
Leave child in location found.
Insulate from ground.
Cover with blanket.
Handle child as little as possible.

Keep child lying flat.
Allow child to shiver.

Do not attempt to rewarm child.
Do not massage child's arms or legs.
Do not elevate legs.
Do not allow child to walk.
Child needs immediate emergency medical care.

Heat-Related Injuries

Most children love the summer and the seemingly endless hours of outdoor play. Adults enjoy having them there for all the health benefits that being outdoors provides. Yet it is important for parents to know that the sun and the heat can be dangerous and occasionally deadly. Use common sense and the recommendations in this section to avoid heat-related injuries, which are caused by overexposure to high temperatures. These injuries can be mild or they can be life-threatening, depending on the degree of heat and the length of time that the child is exposed.

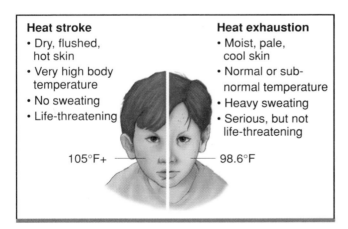

Heat stroke
- Dry, flushed, hot skin
- Very high body temperature
- No sweating
- Life-threatening

105°F+

Heat exhaustion
- Moist, pale, cool skin
- Normal or sub-normal temperature
- Heavy sweating
- Serious, but not life-threatening

98.6°F

Comparison of heat stroke and heat exhaustion

Heat Stroke

Heat stroke is the most severe heat illness and a life-threatening emergency. It occurs when a child is exposed to a very high environmental temperature and can also occur in older children and adults from overexertion in high temperatures. When this happens, the body's heat-regulating ability becomes overwhelmed and ceases to function properly, resulting in an inability to sweat and a dangerously high rise in body temperature. Heat stroke can develop suddenly. Brain, liver and kidney damage, and death can result if the body is not cooled immediately. Hospitalization is always necessary.

The Short Errand Mistake

A pleasant, sunny day of 78°F with a gentle breeze is hardly a day when we think about heat stroke. However, even at this comfortable temperature, the air temperature inside a closed car parked in the sun can reach 120°F in less than 20 minutes. Do not leave a child in a closed car while you run into a store, even for just a few minutes. If you see a child left unattended in a closed car, alert the local police. If the car is unlocked, open the door and check the child.

What to Look For

- Body temperature approaches 106°F or higher. At these temperatures, damage to vital organs, such as the liver, brain, and kidney, can occur in a matter of minutes.
- Skin feels very hot
- Skin feels dry
- Flushed skin (bright red face in light-skinned children)
- Rapid breathing and pulse
- Lethargy
- Confusion, delirium
- Seizure
- Loss of consciousness

What to Do

It is urgent to begin first aid immediately. The longer it takes to get treatment to the child, the more likely it is that there will be serious complications or death.

1. Send someone to call for emergency medical help.
2. Check and monitor the ABCDs and treat, as needed.

3. Move the child into the shade or to an air-conditioned room or car.

4. Remove outer clothing, such as shirt and pants.

5. Begin cooling the child while waiting for emergency medical help to arrive.

   - Place ice packs wrapped in a cloth on the body in areas with abundant blood supply, such as the armpits, groin, and neck. Use this step when the humidity is high, because, in that climate, it can be more effective than spraying and fanning.

   - Gently spray the child with cold water from the garden hose, pour water on the body, or apply cold, wet sheets to the child's head, trunk, and limbs. Do not cover the nose and mouth. Keep the child wet. Continuously fan the child to speed the evaporation of water, which is very effective in reducing temperature. This method is more effective when the humidity is very low, but if you do not have ice in higher humidity, use this method.

6. Have the child seen in an emergency medical facility immediately.

7. Notify the child's parent.

Preventing Heat-Related Injuries

Also see *Sunburn Precautions,* Chapter 6.

- Encourage children to drink cool tap water frequently on hot days, as often as every 2 hours. Fruit juices and popsicles are fine hot weather treats. Also encourage salty snacks, such as pretzels and salty crackers. Do not give salt tablets. Salt is best consumed mixed with water as a drink.

- Avoid vigorous physical activity in direct sun during the midday hours, when temperatures are usually the highest.

- Provide cooling activities, such as a sprinkler or a wading pool.

- Dress children in lightweight and loose-fitting clothing.

- Never leave a child in a closed vehicle in warm weather.

DO NOT

- place a semiconscious or unconscious child in the bathtub or give anything to eat or drink.
- use rubbing alcohol on the child in place of water.
- give aspirin, acetaminophen, or ibuprofen in an attempt to reduce the temperature, because these medications will have no effect.

Heat Exhaustion

Heat exhaustion occurs when the body loses too much water and salt through sweating. In children, it is often the result of prolonged physical activity in high temperatures without pausing to drink enough water. This condition differs from heat stroke in that the child sweats heavily, the body temperature remains normal, and the child's mental status remains clear. Heat exhaustion is less critical than heat stroke, but it requires prompt attention to correct it.

What to Look For

- Body temperature remains normal
- Skin pale and clammy, with heavy sweating
- Fast and weak pulse
- Tiredness and weakness
- Dizziness and feeling faint
- Headache
- Thirst
- Nausea and vomiting
- Muscle cramps

What to Do

1. Move the child to a cool place.

2. Have the child drink a glass of cold water containing ¼ teaspoon of salt. Do not give more than 3 glasses, and give them at 15-minute intervals. If the child is still thirsty, switch to cold water without salt. If you do not have salt available, cold tap water alone is helpful.

3. Sponge the child with cool, wet cloths on the head, face, and trunk.

4. Elevate the feet 8 to 12 inches, but no more.

5. Call the child's parent.

HEAT-RELATED EMERGENCIES

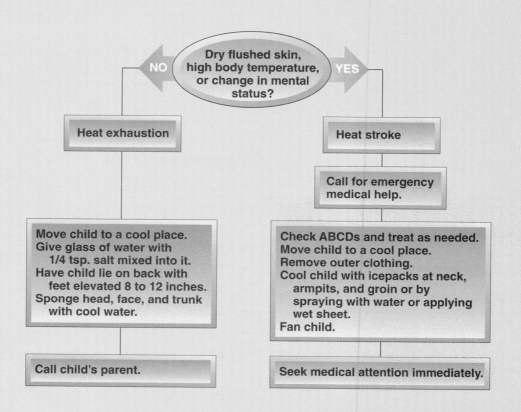

Dry flushed skin, high body temperature, or change in mental status?

NO → Heat exhaustion

Move child to a cool place.
Give glass of water with
   1/4 tsp. salt mixed into it.
Have child lie on back with
   feet elevated 8 to 12 inches.
Sponge head, face, and trunk
   with cool water.

Call child's parent.

YES → Heat stroke

Call for emergency
medical help.

Check ABCDs and treat as needed.
Move child to a cool place.
Remove outer clothing.
Cool child with icepacks at neck,
   armpits, and groin or by
   spraying with water or applying
   wet sheet.
Fan child.

Seek medical attention immediately.

Heat Syncope

A child can easily develop heat syncope from over-exposure to the sun, and it can occur easily in a child who is sensitive to the sun. This condition resembles fainting: the child feels light-headed but does not usually faint. Sometimes, if not treated, heat syncope can lead to heat exhaustion. Minor first aid measures are very effective in treating heat syncope.

What to Look For

- Lightheadedness and dizziness
- Headache
- Nausea

What to Do

1. Have the child lie down in a cool place to rest.
2. If not nauseated, give the child cool water to drink.

The child should begin to feel better within 15 minutes but should not participate in strenuous outdoor activity for the remainder of the day.

Heat Cramps

Heat cramps are painful spasms in muscles that cause a temporary loss of mobility. They are caused by the loss of water and possibly also by the loss of salt through heavy sweating. This results in inadequate circulation to the major leg and abdominal muscles used in exercise or play. The cramping lasts from a few minutes to several hours. Heat cramps are never serious by themselves but can be one of the symptom of heat exhaustion, a more serious heat-related illness.

What to Look For

- Painful cramping that prevents use of the muscle
- Heavy sweating
- Thirst

What to Do

1. Get the child into the most comfortable position possible.
2. Give the child a glass of cold water containing ¼ teaspoon of salt to drink. Do not give more than three glasses and give them at 15-minute intervals. If the child is still thirsty, switch to cold water without salt or give a commercial sports drink but not in large amounts, because the high sugar content slows the absorption of the water in the drink.
3. Rest the muscle. Allow the child to massage or apply gentle continuous direct pressure to help release the cramp. The muscle gradually begins to come out of spasm after 15 minutes or more.
4. Apply ice or a cold pack wrapped in a wet cloth to help relax the muscle.

Drinking one to two glasses of water during the hour before vigorous outdoor play or sports and taking water breaks while exercising can help prevent heat cramps.

Name _____ Course _____ Date _____

1. Circle yes (Y) or no (N) for each statement about treatment for frostbite.

   Y   N   a. Rewarm a frostbitten body part with a heating pad.

   Y   N   b. Massage the frostbitten area to help restore circulation.

   Y   N   c. Wrap frostbitten fingers snugly to-gether to speed rewarming.

   Y   N   d. Rub snow on the frostbitten areas to help restore circulation.

   Y   N   e. Break large blisters that form on frostbitten skin.

2. Circle true (T) or false (F) for the following state-ments about frostbite.

   T   F   a. Adults are more susceptible to frost-bite than children.

   T   F   b. Frostbite is seen most often on hands, noses, and feet.

   T   F   c. Once frostbitten, a body part is more susceptible to future episodes of frostbite.

3. Circle true (T) or false (F) for the following state-ments about hypothermia.

   T   F   a. Hypothermia occurs only in the winter.

   T   F   b. Shivering is the body's way to in-crease its temperature.

   T   F   c. Wind can increase heat loss from the body.

   T   F   d. Gloves keep fingers warmer than mittens.

4. Match the heat-related condition to the signs or symptoms.
   HS (Heat stroke)
   HE (Heat exhaustion)

   ____ a. Can be sudden and life-threatening

   ____ b. Flushed skin

   ____ c. Heavy sweating

   ____ d. Normal body temperature

   ____ e. Skin feels very hot

5. You spot an infant in the back seat of a closed but unlocked car in a parking lot outside of a shop-ping area on a hot summer day. The child appears to be sleeping. What steps might you take?

   a. _____

   b. _____

   c. _____

6. One hot summer day, four-year-old Ricky com-plains that his head hurts and he feels sick to his stomach after playing vigorously in your back yard for several hours. What should you do?

   a. _____

   b. _____

   c. _____

7. What might you have done to help prevent Ricky's problem in question 6?

   _____

8. Five-year-old Kristen comes inside after riding her bike late in the afternoon on a hot day. She is holding her left lower leg. She is crying in pain but says that she did not fall. She says her leg muscle just started to hurt. What should you do?

   a. _____

   b. _____

   c. _____

CHAPTER 12

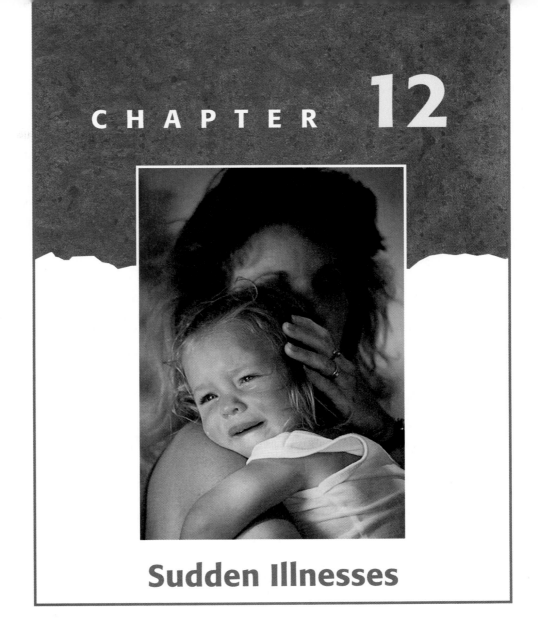

Sudden Illnesses

Croup

Croup is an acute swelling of the vocal cords caused by a viral infection and is common in infants and young children. It is not a disease itself but a group of respiratory symptoms that lasts for 3 to 5 days and can usually be treated at home.

An attack of croup typically occurs suddenly and at night. The child wakes with a hoarse, barking cough and difficulty breathing. The child has flaring nostrils and works very hard to breathe, sometimes using muscles of the neck and abdomen. Often the nose and lips have a blue or gray discoloration. Usually there is no fever.

What to Do

1. Take the child, along with a favorite book or stuffed animal, into the bathroom and close the door. Hold the child on your lap outside the shower and turn on the hot shower to produce misting in the room. This misting helps to decrease the swelling of air passages. Holding the child close to a

cool mist vaporizer in the bedroom produces the same effect. The child's breathing should show signs of improvement in 10 to 15 minutes.

2. If breathing difficulty recurs or if the child continues to have difficulty breathing after this treatment, call the child's health care provider. He or she might want to see the child. If it is the middle of the night, you will be instructed to take the child to an emergency medical facility. If traveling by car, open the windows to allow the child to breathe cold air. This also helps to decrease swelling and to make breathing easier.

Dehydration

Dehydration is an excessive loss of fluids from the body, which occurs when the total amount of water lost through sweating, urination, diarrhea, and vomiting is greater than what is taken in. Illnesses such as fever, vomiting, diarrhea, and heat exhaustion are especially worrisome in infants and young children because dehydration can occur easily. A child with severe dehydration must be hospitalized to receive intravenous fluids.

When a child is sick, offer frequent sips of clear fluids to prevent dehydration. See clear fluid suggestions in *Vomiting,* in Chapter 16. Even the most diligent parent or child care provider sometimes has difficulty getting a child to drink, if the child has pain in the throat from problems such as chicken pox blisters or is too weak from an illness to drink.

What to Look For

- A decreased amount of urine that is deep gold in color and has a strong odor, because it is more concentrated
- No tears when crying
- Dry, cracked lips with little or no salivation
- Irritability or fussiness
- Dry skin; no sweating
- Sunken eyes
- Listlessness, sleepiness
- Poor skin turgor—to determine this, lightly pull up a fold of skin and release it. Skin with poor turgor returns slowly to normal position or remains "tented."

- A sunken fontanel (soft spot) in an infant under the approximate age of 1 year

What to Do

1. Call the parent if the child shows any signs of dehydration. A parent should contact the health care provider for advice on how to correct the problem. The health care provider might want to examine the child or might recommend that the child be taken to an emergency medical facility.

2. The child's health care provider should be contacted if the child:
    - Has been unable to drink for several hours as a result of illness, especially an infant under the age of 6 months
    - Has had several episodes of vomiting and diarrhea
    - Has had watery diarrhea for 2 to 3 days

Fainting

Fainting is a sudden and temporary loss of consciousness caused by a brief lack of blood and oxygen to the brain. Fainting is not caused by an injury; it is a nervous system reaction to such situations as fear, pain, or a strong emotional upset. Occasionally, prolonged standing, especially in a warm environment, results in fainting.

What to Look For

Warning signs and symptoms that a child is about to faint include:

- Lightheadedness and dizziness
- Seeing spots or unusual images
- Nausea
- Pale skin color
- Sweating

What to Do

1. Lay the child on the back to prevent falling. If the child has already fainted, position the child on the back.

2. Elevate the legs 8 to 12 inches to increase blood flow to the brain, possibly avoiding fainting altogether.

3. Loosen tight-fitting clothing.

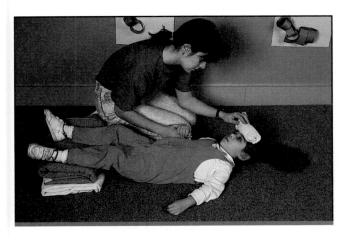

Positioning and care for a child who has fainted

4. Apply a cool, wet cloth to the face.

5. If vomiting begins, position the child on the left side in the recovery position to prevent choking and to prevent vomit from entering the lungs.

6. Check for injuries that might have occurred from falling.

DO NOT

- **give anything to eat or drink until the child is well enough to continue with a normal routine.**
- **use smelling salts or ammonia, because they irritate the lining of the nose and breathing passageways.**
- **slap the face in an attempt to revive the child.**

A child who has fainted recovers quickly, often in 1 to 2 minutes. Fainting is generally not serious and, in children, can usually be traced to a triggering event. You should call for emergency medical help if the child fails to recover from fainting and remains unconscious. The child should be seen by a health care provider if the child has repeated attacks of fainting for no apparent reason.

Some young children cause themselves to faint by holding their breath. These breath-holding spells are often caused by frustration or anger and sometimes by fear. Commonly, uncontrolled crying is followed by breath holding until the child loses consciousness. The child begins to breathe spontaneously after fainting and regains consciousness within several seconds. There is no specific treatment, and the episodes disappear as the child matures. A parent might want to discuss the problem with the child's health care provider.

Near-Drowning

Drowning is a leading cause of injury resulting in death among children. More than one half of all drownings happen to children ages 5 and under. Drowning can be a silent killer, and it can happen quickly. Equally sad are the near-drowning victims who survive but suffer brain damage and a reduced quality of life. Near-drowning refers to surviving a prolonged period of time under water without oxygen.

A drowning or a near-drowning can occur in any body of water in which the nose and mouth of a child can be submerged. Besides the obvious large bodies of deep water, drownings can also occur in toilets, bath tubs, sinks, water buckets, fish tanks, and wading pools with only inches of water.

What to Do

1. Shout for help and send someone to call for emergency medical help.

2. Rescue the child from the water. If you suspect that a spinal injury has occurred because the child is unconscious or is injured after a dive, keep the head, neck, and spine straight. To do this, float the child onto a large full-body board and lift the child out of the water gently, supporting the head and neck.

3. Establish consciousness, check the ABCDs and treat as needed. If you are alone and must perform either rescue breathing or CPR, do so for 1 minute before stopping to call for emergency medical help yourself.

4. If the child vomits, which is likely after a near-drowning, roll the child onto the left side as one unit to avoid twisting the neck and spine. This position allows for vomit to drain and keeps the airway open.

Although infrequent, successful rescues have occurred after prolonged submersions in cold water. This is because the body's oxygen requirement is reduced in cold water, making it possible for the brain to survive longer without oxygen than the standard 4 to 6 minutes. Read about safety for children in and around all bodies of water in *Water Safety*, Chapter 17.

Water Rescues

If a child is in trouble in the water, adults should only attempt rescues that they are sure they can perform safely and that they have been trained to perform. Rescuers should never jeopardize themselves and risk becoming an additional victim. The phrase "Reach, throw, row, go " tells you the order in which to try methods to reach a child struggling in water. The following are rescue methods that can be used to attempt to reach a child in the water:

- Reach a conscious, struggling child from the shore with a branch, pole, rope, or towel.

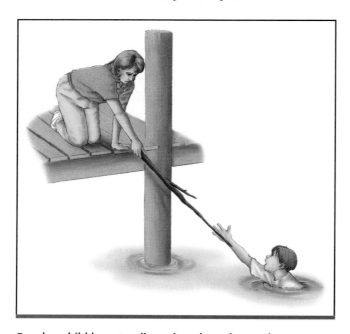

Reach a child by extending a long branch or pole.

- If beyond this reach, throw anything that floats, such as a styrofoam kick board, an inner tube, a life jacket, an empty cooler, or other airtight

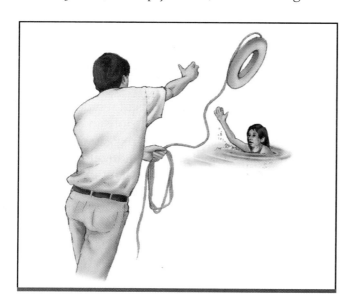

Throw an object that floats.

plastic container. Tie a rope to it if one is available.

- Use a boat if one is available to rescue a child who is far off shore. Pull the child into the boat over the end of the boat to avoid tipping. Be sure that you are wearing a life jacket.

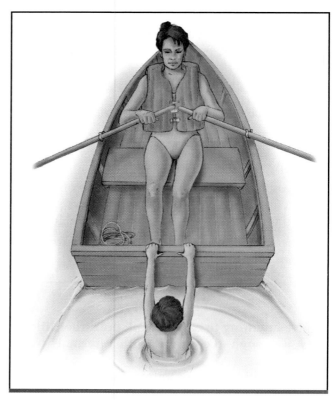

Use a boat to reach a child far off shore.

- Swim to a child only if you are trained in how to do this form of rescue. Take a towel to extend to the child or an object that floats for

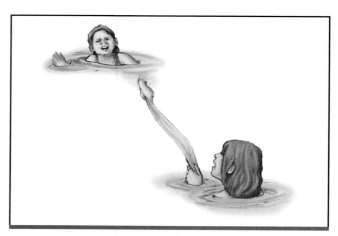

If swimming to the child is the only option, extend a towel or other object to avoid having the child grab you.

the child to grasp. For the safety of each of you, do not let the child grab you.

Ice Rescues

For a child who has fallen through ice, extend a lightweight pole or branch or throw a rope to the child. Have someone grab your waist to stabilize you. As the child is pulled out, tell the child to spread the arms over the ice to distribute weight evenly. If you have nothing to extend and there are enough people present, try to reach the child by forming a human chain. Lie flat on the ice and grab the ankles of the person ahead of you to distribute weight evenly.

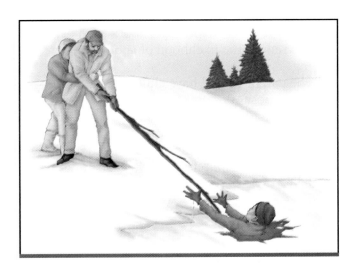

Extend a long object or rope to reach the child.

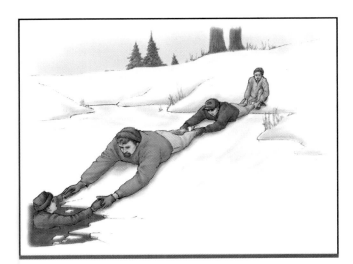

If an object is not available, make a human chain to distribute weight evenly.

Seizures

A seizure, or convulsion, is a disturbance in the electrical impulses of the brain. Such disturbances result in a variety of body responses. These range from the very mild, such as a few moments of staring, to the more severe collapse on the floor with loss of consciousness and the strong shaking of large voluntary muscles. Causes of seizures, other than brain abnormality and genetic factors include: high fever, head injury, drug overdose or reaction, serious illness, and poisoning. A person who experiences a seizure for the first time should always receive immediate emergency medical care.

Sometimes a specific cause of the seizure can be identified, but more commonly, the cause remains unknown. Even without knowing the exact cause, a health care provider can usually treat the child with medication to control the seizures or reduce their frequency.

When this type of seizure is about to happen, an older and experienced child might be able to recognize specific symptoms, known as an "aura." This is an internal warning system, which can be a noise, visual change, funny taste, numbness, or other feeling that causes the child to know that a seizure is about to occur. Other children experience no aura or cannot recognize it as such and do not know that the seizure is about to start.

The most easily recognizable seizure, and one for which first aid care is helpful, involves the entire body and is called a grand mal seizure.

What to Look For

- Loss of consciousness
- Breathing stops temporarily
- Rigid body with jerking and shaking movements
- Neck and back arch
- Eyes roll back
- Increased saliva production causing drooling or foaming at the mouth
- Incontinence of urine or stool

The uncontrolled movements of a child having a seizure can be frightening to watch. Reassure other children who may be watching. A seizure must run its course. There is nothing you can do to interrupt it or stop it.

What to Do

1. Position the child on the left side in the recovery position to allow saliva to drain and to keep the tongue from blocking the airway.

2. Move toys and furniture out of the way so that the child is not injured during the seizure.

3. Slide the palm of your hand or a folded towel under the child's head and allow the head to bump against this cushion rather than the floor.

4. Time the seizure and observe the body parts affected. A seizure might seem to last longer than it actually does, especially if you are frightened. Your detailed description is important to the child's health care provider.

5. Let the child rest in the recovery position after the seizure. Recovery from a seizure is slow and the child will sleep or be drowsy for a while.

6. Have the child seen in an emergency medical facility for a first seizure. Check for a medical alert tag that might identify a seizure disorder. If this is a second febrile seizure or if the child has a known seizure disorder, call the child's health care provider. The child's health care provider or parent should let you know how to treat subsequent seizures.

DO NOT

- force anything between the child's teeth.
- restrain the child's movements.
- give anything to eat or drink until the child is fully alert.

Febrile Seizures

In a small percentage of children, a rapid rise in fever can cause a grand mal seizure. A febrile seizure is not related to a chronic seizure disorder and has no effect on the child's neurologic development or brain function.

A febrile seizure rarely occurs in children under the age of 6 months and is most common between the ages of 18 months and 3 years. It seldom occurs in children over the age of 6 years. A child who has experienced a febrile seizure is more likely to have another one.

Treat a febrile seizure as you would any grand mal seizure. A child who has a febrile seizure for the first time should be seen in an emergency medical facility immediately. If the child has experienced a febrile seizure the parent should speak with the child's health care provider about what can be done to reduce the likelihood of another seizure occurring.

The parent should have children's acetaminophen suppositories on hand. They are an easy way to get fever-reducing medicine into a child who is too ill to swallow or to be cooperative or is nauseated or vomiting. They can be purchased over-the-counter but are kept refrigerated, so one must ask for them.

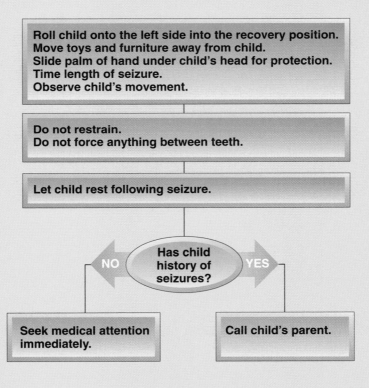

Roll child onto the left side into the recovery position.
Move toys and furniture away from child.
Slide palm of hand under child's head for protection.
Time length of seizure.
Observe child's movement.

Do not restrain.
Do not force anything between teeth.

Let child rest following seizure.

Has child history of seizures?

NO

YES

Seek medical attention immediately.

Call child's parent.

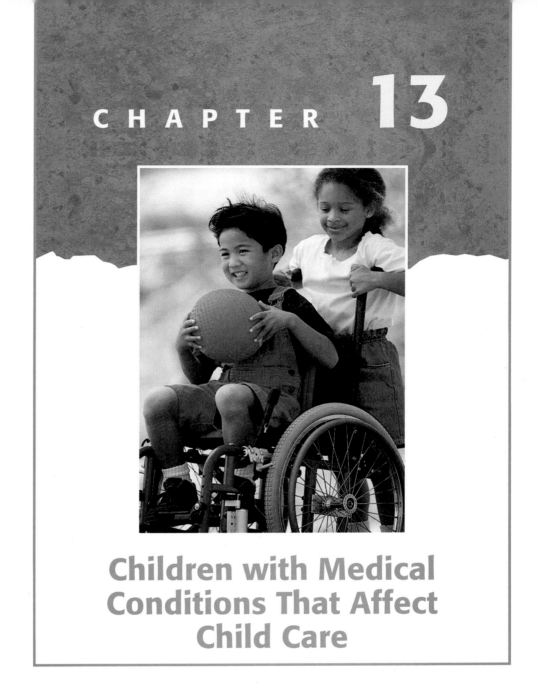

CHAPTER 13

Children with Medical Conditions That Affect Child Care

Asthma

Asthma is a common chronic disease of childhood, affecting more than 5 million children. According to the American Lung Association, asthma is on the increase in both children and adults, as a result of increased exposure to environmental pollutants and irritants. In fact, the number of Americans who have asthma has increased by 60% since the early 1980s.

The sporadic breathing difficulties that a child with asthma experiences are often called "attacks." During these attacks, the lining of the airways throughout the lungs swell, narrow, and partially obstruct. The normal production of mucus increases, further narrowing the airway. Additionally, the muscles surrounding the chest tighten, making breathing difficult. Asthma attacks vary in length and intensity. Some children experience an annoying cough lasting for several days, weeks, or even months. Other children have a sudden attack with breathing difficulty so severe that they cannot complete a sentence without taking a breath.

In some children, asthma is so mild that it is termed "hidden," and the disease can go unnoticed. Commonly, these children have more frequent upper respiratory infections and mild coughs. Their inability to take long, deep breaths often prohibits them from participating in vigorous activity.

Asthma Triggers

Children with asthma have difficulty breathing when exposed to various allergens and other nonallergic

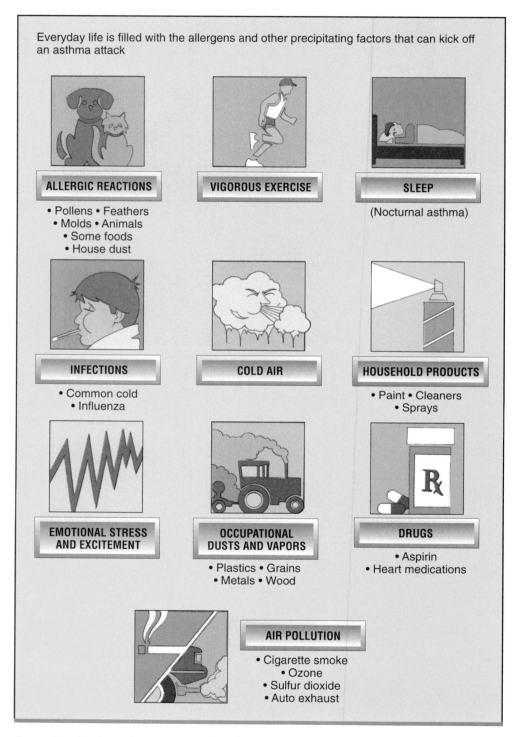

Everyday life is filled with the allergens and other precipitating factors that can kick off an asthma attack

ALLERGIC REACTIONS
• Pollens • Feathers
• Molds • Animals
• Some foods
• House dust

VIGOROUS EXERCISE

SLEEP
(Nocturnal asthma)

INFECTIONS
• Common cold
• Influenza

COLD AIR

HOUSEHOLD PRODUCTS
• Paint • Cleaners
• Sprays

EMOTIONAL STRESS AND EXCITEMENT

OCCUPATIONAL DUSTS AND VAPORS
• Plastics • Grains
• Metals • Wood

DRUGS
• Aspirin
• Heart medications

AIR POLLUTION
• Cigarette smoke
• Ozone
• Sulfur dioxide
• Auto exhaust

Source: American Lung Association®—The "Christmas Seal People.®"

irritants. These substances are called "asthma triggers." Common asthma triggers are:

- **Infections.** Upper respiratory infections, such as the common cold, can trigger an episode of asthma.

- **Allergens.** Common substances that trigger allergic responses are dust, mold, pollen, feathers, and animal dander. Additionally, allergies to certain medications and, infrequently, allergies to foods such as eggs, milk, grains, and chocolate can cause an asthma attack.

- **Irritants.** These substances cause coughing, a runny nose, watery eyes, and tightness in the muscles of the chest. Air pollution and second-hand cigarette smoke are major irritants to a child with asthma.

- **Exercise.** According to the American Lung Association, vigorous exercise such as running can trigger an episode of asthma in more than 80% of children with the disease. The exercise that is least likely to stimulate an episode of asthma is swimming. Asthma attacks resulting from exercise are often controlled with medication taken before the activity.

- **Weather.** Changes in the weather can stimulate an asthma attack in a child with the disease. Windy days in the spring and fall stir up pollens and dust in the air, and the dry, cold winter air can irritate the lining of the airways.

- **Emotion.** Although psychological factors are not a cause of asthma, they can influence the course of an attack. Emotional stress or the extreme excitement of laughing or crying in a child who has asthma can result in rapid breathing and an episode of wheezing. Also, a child who is experiencing tightness in the chest and breathing difficulties feels anxious. The anxiety is worsened if the parent appears anxious, too.

Children must be taught which allergic substances and irritants trigger their asthma attacks and how to avoid them, so that they can start sharing the responsibility for monitoring and managing the particulars of their health condition.

What to Look For

- **Coughing.** Coughing is the body's response to an irritation in the airway. A child with asthma eventually learns how to cough up mucus to clear the airway. Often, coughing is more frequent at night.

- **Wheezing.** The wheezing breath sound is caused by narrowing of the airway and is heard on both inhalation and exhalation.

- **Chest tightness and shortness of breath.** This is especially common following vigorous exercise. During a severe attack, the child's nostrils flare and abdominal and neck muscles are used to help pull air into the lungs.

- **Increased pulse and respiratory rate.** These increase in response to the need to eliminate a buildup of carbon dioxide.

What to Do

1. Have the child sit in a quiet area.
2. Give asthma medication as prescribed by the child's health care provider.
3. Give the child plenty of clear fluids to help thin the mucus in the lungs and make it easier for the child to cough up the secretions.
4. Keep the child at rest until the child is breathing comfortably and feels better.

DO NOT

- **give asthma medication more often than prescribed.**

Call the child's parent to contact the health care provider if:

- The child is unable to speak easily.
- The child has flaring nostrils and is working very hard to breathe, using the muscles of the neck and abdomen.
- The child's lips have a blue or gray discoloration.
- The child does not improve within 30 to 45 minutes after taking the medication.

Diabetic Emergencies

Diabetes is a chronic illness that affects both adults and children and interferes with their ability to produce insulin and regulate blood sugar. Uncontrolled, diabetes can produce two separate medical crises: hypoglycemia and hyperglycemia.

ASTHMA

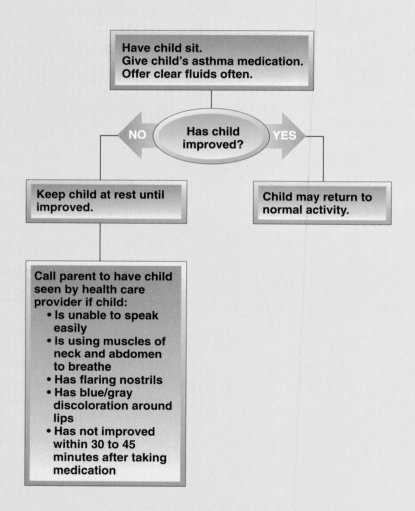

Have child sit.
Give child's asthma medication.
Offer clear fluids often.

Has child improved?

NO

YES

Keep child at rest until improved.

Child may return to normal activity.

Call parent to have child seen by health care provider if child:
- Is unable to speak easily
- Is using muscles of neck and abdomen to breathe
- Has flaring nostrils
- Has blue/gray discoloration around lips
- Has not improved within 30 to 45 minutes after taking medication

Hypoglycemia

Hypoglycemia is an abnormally low level of glucose, or sugar, in the blood. In the diabetic child, it means that there is too much insulin and not enough glucose circulating in the bloodstream. This causes an insulin reaction, or insulin shock, which comes on quickly and must be treated immediately. It is the most common medical emergency for a child with diabetes and can be life-threatening if ignored.

In a nondiabetic child, insulin levels rise and fall automatically in response to meals and activity level. But children with diabetes cannot produce insulin, so they must receive one or two insulin injections each day and then must regulate meals and activity so that there is always enough glucose in the blood to balance the amount of insulin there.

If the blood glucose level dips too low, hypoglycemia occurs. This can happen if the child does not eat enough food, waits too long for a snack or meal, is unusually physically active, or receives too much insulin.

For a diabetic child, an important part of being in control of the disease is learning to recognize the early sensations that occur when an insulin reaction is about to happen. A trained child knows the circumstances in which a reaction can happen, knows to recognize its onset, and knows to immediately consume a piece of candy, a glass of orange juice, or another quick source of sugar, so that the blood sugar rapidly returns to a proper level and the insulin reaction is avoided altogether. In a young diabetic child or a newly diagnosed diabetic child, early recognition of these signs is not always possible.

What to Look For

Early signs (which appear suddenly):

- Hunger
- Anger, irritability
- Weakness
- Trembling
- Sweating
- Dizziness

Later signs:

- Drowsiness
- Impaired thinking and coordination
- Confusion
- Loss of consciousness

What to Do

1. Give the child a fast-acting sugar, such as table sugar, a sugar cube, honey, cake frosting, candy, or orange juice, if the child is alert enough to swallow. The child should feel better in 10 to 15 minutes. Check whether a meal or snack was missed.

2. If there is no improvement in 15 minutes, give the same amount of sugar again and call the child's parent or health care provider.

3. If a child with diabetes is found unconscious, place a small amount of table sugar or cake frosting under the tongue. Check and monitor the ABCDs and treat accordingly. Position the child on the left side in the recovery position. Call for emergency medical help.

DO NOT

- give the child a diet soft drink, because it does not contain any sugar.
- give sugar in a liquid form, such as juice or a soft drink, to an unconscious diabetic child.

Hyperglycemia

Hyperglycemia occurs when there is too much glucose and not enough insulin in the bloodstream. Persistent high blood sugar levels impair circulation, damage blood vessels and organs, and make the child particularly susceptible to infection.

Hyperglycemia occurs in a child with an undiagnosed case of diabetes. It can also occur in a child who has diabetes, indicating either an illness or a need to readjust insulin dose or food intake. Hyperglycemia is not an immediate medical emergency in terms of first aid. It can take several days or even weeks to recognize the signs and symptoms.

What to Look For

- Excessive thirst
- Excessive hunger
- Excessive urination
- Fruity breath odor
- Sudden unexplained weight loss
- Weakness
- Overly tired and irritable

DIABETIC EMERGENCY: HYPOGLYCEMIA (INSULIN REACTION)

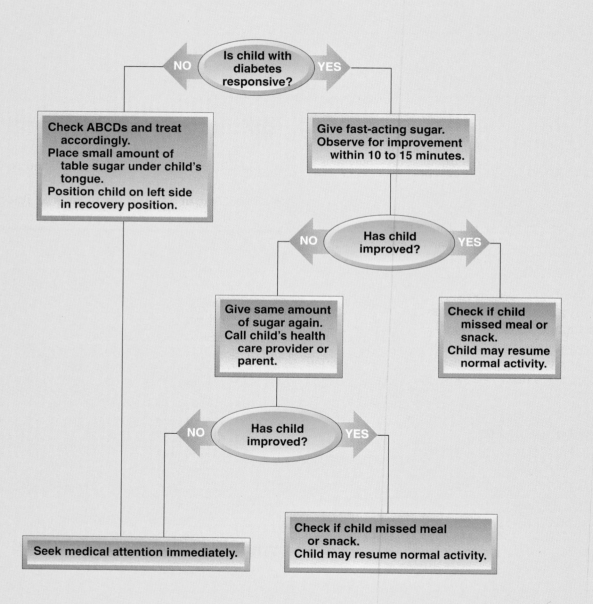

Is child with diabetes responsive?

NO → Check ABCDs and treat accordingly.
Place small amount of table sugar under child's tongue.
Position child on left side in recovery position.

YES → Give fast-acting sugar. Observe for improvement within 10 to 15 minutes.

Has child improved?

NO → Give same amount of sugar again. Call child's health care provider or parent.

YES → Check if child missed meal or snack. Child may resume normal activity.

Has child improved?

NO → Seek medical attention immediately.

YES → Check if child missed meal or snack. Child may resume normal activity.

During normal digestion, much of the food we eat is broken down into a sugar, called glucose, which the body uses as fuel for the cells. Glucose enters the bloodstream, where it is transported from the blood into the cells with the help of insulin. The pancreas, an organ of digestion, normally produces insulin whenever food is eaten and releases that insulin into the blood. The insulin then attaches to the glucose and transports it from the blood into the cells to nourish them. Without insulin, the glucose is available in the bloodstream but is unable to get to those cells. The cells do not get nourished, and the body begins to starve. This leads to weakness and fatigue. In addition, the high level of glucose in the blood makes the body particularly susceptible to infection.

The accumulating glucose is filtered out of the blood by the kidneys and spills into the urine. This process requires extra water, which produces *thirst*. The glucose in the urine is lost, leaving the body unnourished, and producing insatiable *hunger*. The body turns to its supply of stored fat to make energy, which produces significant *weight loss*. These are the three telling signs of the development of diabetes—weight loss, thirst, and hunger.

Unlike glucose, fat does not require insulin to transport it into the cells. However, in using fats for energy, the body produces unhealthy wastes call ketones. A buildup of ketones in the blood results in a condition known as ketoacidosis. If ketoacidosis is left untreated, it can lead to coma and death. The buildup of ketones in the blood produces a *fruity odor to the breath,* which is another indicator of developing diabetes.

- Bed-wetting
- Drowsiness in advanced cases

A child who does not have diabetes can show one or two of these symptoms occasionally. But a child with developing or poorly controlled diabetes shows several of these signs persistently. Often it is the sudden onset of bed-wetting and unexplained weight loss that causes the parent to take the child to a health care provider.

What to Do

If a child has some of the above signs and symptoms consistently, he or she should be seen by a health care provider. Untreated, hyperglycemia results in further deterioration of the child's health. If a child's hyperglycemia is allowed to reach an advanced stage in which drowsiness or even loss of consciousness occurs, the child will need emergency medical care and a period of hospitalization.

Where does diabetes come from? Childhood diabetes has no clearly evident source. All people can inherit genes that make them more susceptible to the risk of developing type I diabetes. A gene is a tiny part of a chromosome that determines a range of characteristics for the child—from sex and eye color to some health problems. However, genes might need to be stimulated by a viral illness and an immune system problem for diabetes to develop.

Could the child's diabetes have been prevented? No. There are some stresses, such as illness or infection, that might cause the diabetes to show its presence earlier in life, but diabetes cannot be prevented.

Does eating a lot of sweets cause diabetes? No. Despite what people think, there is no evidence to suggest that this is true. You will not use up your body's supply of insulin eating too many sweet foods. Eating a diet high in sweets can contribute to dental cavities, childhood obesity, and poor nutrition. None of these are desirable, but they are not causes of diabetes.

Will diabetes go away after insulin treatment and leave the child cured? No. At present, there is no cure for diabetes. It is a lifelong, controllable health condition. Once controlled and then well managed, the child develops physically, emotionally, and socially.

Is diabetes contagious? No. You cannot catch diabetes from another individual. Activities such as sharing a drinking cup or a piece of food, or touching blood or saliva, are not ways of developing diabetes.

HIV in a Child Care Setting

HIV is one of the largest health problems that the world faces today. The Centers for Disease Control estimates that in the United States alone, more than 1 million people are infected with HIV (human immunodeficiency virus), which causes AIDS (acquired

Special Considerations for a Child with Diabetes

Diabetes is a lifelong illness that affects every aspect of the child's life. Constant daily insulin injections and testing blood for glucose, as well as following lifelong diet restrictions make diabetes a demanding disease.

The delicate balance between glucose and insulin levels in the blood is affected by the child's diet, physical activity, illness, and stress. Controlling the disease successfully in a child requires a team effort from the child, parents, health care provider, and child care provider.

Diet. A child with diabetes needs a diet of foods that are high in nutritional value and low in concentrated sugar. It is essential for meals and snacks to be eaten at regular intervals to maintain the balance between glucose and insulin. Most children with diabetes need a morning and afternoon snack. Parents give child care providers specific instructions about their child's diet. A child care provider is responsible for making snacks and mealtimes pleasant.

Parties and holiday celebrations present special problems when restricted foods are plentiful in the classroom. Food exchanges and substitutions that allow a child to eat special treats are occasionally permitted but should be discussed with the child's parent. *Physical Activity.* Most children with diabetes should be encouraged to participate fully in all activities of the child care center or school. Parents should provide information on any necessary restrictions. Strenuous activity can upset the balance between insulin and glucose in the blood and cause insulin shock. Do not restrict the child's activities for fear of insulin shock; instead, understand that the child's diet can be adjusted to ensure that the child has the additional energy necessary for energetic play or a special activity. *Illness and Stress.* Illnesses and stress increase the demands on the body because they upset the balance between glucose and insulin. A child care provider must be especially watchful of a child with diabetes who is ill or stressed.

Diabetic Emergency Summary Chart

	Hyperglycemia	Hypoglycemia (insulin reaction)
Cause	Too much sugar and too little insulin	Too little sugar and too much insulin
Develops	Slowly, over a period of days or weeks	Suddenly, within seconds or minutes
Signs	Persistent hunger Persistent thirst Frequent urination Dry mouth and skin Unexplained weight loss Stomachache	Trembling Dizziness Weakness Sweating Irritability Hunger Headache
Advanced Signs	Flushed skin Vomiting Abdominal pain Fruity breath Difficulty breathing Loss of consciousness	Anger Confusion Blurred vision Impaired thinking and confusion Loss of consciousness
Treatment	Insulin	Give sugar in form of table sugar, honey, regular soft drinks, frosting
Correctable	Over a period of days or weeks in a hospital	Usually at home or child care center within 15 minutes of eating sugar

immune deficiency syndrome). Initially, HIV lives within the body for months or years before the signs and symptoms of AIDS appear. In time, the virus begins to destroy the immune system, making the body susceptible to chronic infections that become increasingly difficult to fight. Illnesses that might be minor to a person with a healthy immune system, such as chicken pox and flu, can become dangerous and even life threatening to a person with HIV.

People who have HIV in their blood but have a healthy immune system are able to fight infection. Healthy HIV-infected persons can still transmit the virus to others, even though they have no symptoms of the disease and might not know they are infected. There is presently no vaccine or cure for HIV.

HIV is found in infected blood, semen, vaginal secretions, and breast milk. The virus is also present in other body fluids, including saliva, tears, perspiration, urine, and feces, but not in concentrations high enough to transmit the disease. However, the virus can be spread through any of these fluids if they contain HIV-infected blood, even in microscopic amounts.

HIV is a fragile virus and is not easily transmitted from person to person through ordinary, everyday activities. Some behaviors have been identified as high risk for transmitting HIV. These include unprotected sexual activity, sharing needles and syringes for drug use, body piercing and tattooing with uncleaned needles, sharing a toothbrush or a razor, and allowing blood or any body fluid containing even microscopic amounts of blood to come in contact with an open cut or sore, no matter how small the opening or where it is located.

HIV can be transmitted from an HIV-infected mother to her unborn child. Some children born to HIV-infected mothers initially test positive for HIV. Many of these children, however, will lose the HIV antibody as they naturally lose other maternal antibodies during their first year of life. Therefore, a positive test for HIV shortly after birth is not a reliable indicator that the child actually is infected with HIV. In rare cases, HIV has been transmitted to a healthy infant by an HIV-infected mother through her breast milk.

HIV can also be transmitted through a transfusion of blood or blood products contaminated with the virus. However, this risk is very small because all blood and blood products are now carefully screened for HIV. There is *no* risk of becoming infected with HIV when donating blood.

HIV is *not* spread through such ordinary everyday activities as:

- Hugging
- Dry kissing
- Holding hands
- Sneezing or coughing
- Cooking
- Sharing foods
- Using public telephones
- Using public restrooms
- Using public swimming pools
- Touching money, furniture, doorknobs, etc.
- Using playground equipment and sandboxes
- Sharing books and toys
- Playing with a cat or a dog
- Being bitten by a mosquito
- Having an ear pierced by a commercial hand-held puncher

According to the U.S. Surgeon General, there are no documented cases of HIV transmission from one child to another in a school, child care, or foster care setting. Transmission of the virus in these settings would require the unlikely contact of one child's open cut with the blood or other body fluids of an HIV-infected child.

The number of children with HIV in child care in the United States is small but growing. However, for every child known to have HIV, there are other HIV-infected children whose health care providers, parents, and child care provider do not yet know that the virus is present. It is therefore essential for all child care providers to know how to handle body fluids correctly. Child care providers must:

- Wear disposable gloves when giving first aid for a cut or wound, changing diapers, and handling or wiping up body fluids, such as blood and vomit. If gloves are not immediately available when first aid is necessary, use another barrier. Examples of other barriers are several thick gauze pads, a clean dish towel, or a cloth diaper. Plastic wrap or a plastic bag placed over the gauze or cloth increases the effectiveness of these barriers.

- Use disposable diapers. Soiled diapers should be folded with the soiled side inward and placed in a double-lined, covered diaper pail.

- Clean blood and other fluids off all surfaces with a solution of ten parts water to one part bleach. Allow this solution to air dry.
- Wash your hands vigorously with soap and warm water after removing disposable gloves.

Handle *all* body fluids for *all* children in this manner at *all* times.

Information contained in a child's medical record is confidential. A child care center must protect the privacy of a child who is infected with HIV by limiting the number of people who have knowledge of the child's condition. Each case of a child with HIV in a child care setting must be evaluated individually to determine how the center can best provide for the needs of the child. Decisions should be made jointly by the child's parent, health care provider, and child care center director and should be reevaluated periodically.

The problem of HIV infections and AIDS in the United States is growing at an alarming rate and child care providers continue to see increased numbers of children with HIV. Child care providers must take responsibility for keeping up with new information on HIV and AIDS. Contact your local public health department or state AIDS information office, or call the National AIDS Information Hot Line (toll free): 1-800-342-AIDS. For Spanish-speaking persons, call Linea Nacional de SIDA (toll free): 1-800-344-SIDA.

Children with Developmental and Medical Disabilities

In recent years there has been a new direction in American education in which children who have disabilities are educated in their neighborhood schools alongside their typical peers in general education classrooms. This kind of interaction is often termed, "inclusion" or "integration." There is significant data, as well as thousands of anecdotal stories, demonstrating success for all students by including those with disabilities along with their nondisabled friends. In addition, children whose conditions require the care of a nurse are also finding a place in general education classrooms. Examples of such a child, termed "medically fragile," are a child with a tracheostomy, a feeding tube, a need for oxygen, or an impaired immune system or other life-threatening illness.

It is hoped that typical children who are accustomed to being with children with disabilities as a

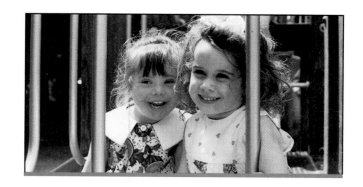

natural part of school life will help eliminate the misconception that people with disabilites are inferior, unapproachable, and nothing like them. After all, any one of us or any one of our children could become disabled or seriously ill, either temporarily or permanently, at any time.

Advocates for children who have disabilities feel that this type of education is the next step for breaking down social barriers in a civilized society. More than just being the right thing to do, however, it is also the law that these children have a place in general education classrooms that meets their unique needs. The Education of the Handicapped Act, Public Law 94-142, was passed by Congress in 1975, amended in 1986, and amended again in 1990 along with a name change to IDEA, which stands for Individuals with Disabilities Education Act. A free public education is a right, not a privilege, for all Americans, and those who have a disability are not to be discounted.

Beginning at the age of 3, all children with disabilities must receive services from state agencies and school systems. Infants and toddlers are also provided for in an early intervention component of the law. This identifies children from birth to age 3 who are experiencing developmental delays and provides supports and services for them and their families to assist in their development.

The inclusion of preschool children who have disabilities in typical child care centers and nursery schools is the beginning of the educational and social experience for these children. In many of today's child care centers and nursery schools, there are children who use wheelchairs, walkers, and other adaptive equipment, children with visual and hearing impairments, and children who have a myriad of medical problems, developmental delays, and behavioral disabilities. To adequately support them in the child care or school setting, children with disabilities might also receive services from special education teachers or teaching assistants, nurses, physical therapists, occupational therapists, adaptive physical therapists, or speech therapists.

Children with special needs should be treated like other children as much as possible. Being held to many of the same standards as the other children in their class helps them gain self-confidence and independence. It also helps to correct some of the incorrect assumptions that adults and other children sometimes make about them and their capabilities.

As a child care provider, you might, at times, feel frustrated and even sad for the child's situation, but it is important not to feel pity. Allowing yourself to feel pity lowers your expectations for the child, and this lowered set of standards is recognized by the child and negatively affects progress and overall success. As you get to know the child, you learn where the child's strengths lie. Expecting the child to conform to as many rules as possible, participate with the others, and attempt new experiences helps him or her have a positive preschool experience. A child with a disability is often a happy child who does not live in a constant state of frustration, is often just as healthy overall as a typical child, and feels all the same emotions as the other children.

Generally, when a child with special needs attends a child care center, the center's staff receives instructions about special circumstances that might need attention, such as toileting, eating, or special precautions concerning outdoor play activities. In many instances, you need to make special arrangements or adaptations to help the child participate. Professional therapists often involve center staff in therapy sessions and encourage typical children to be part of a group session to help promote activities with peers in conjunction with the benefits of the particular therapy.

Often, parents are strong advocates for their children. They are usually your best resource in terms of describing what the child's strengths and needs are and in finding activities that help you discover where the child excels and where the child is most challenged. They can help you determine how best to include the child in a circle of friends within the child care center.

Nondisabled children in the child care center adjust easily to having a friend with a special need. Young children do not have opinions or prejudices concerning disabilities, only healthy curiosity. Children at this age do not hesitate to speak what is on their minds, and they ask simple questions that can be answered fairly easily. Having their questions answered in a matter-of-fact way allows the friendship between them and the disabled child to develop naturally. Young children should be encouraged to ask questions about disabilities and should never be made to feel embarrassed or wrong for asking a question. Questions like, "Why are you in a wheelchair?," "Why do you wear a helmet?," "Why does that lady come to see you?," or "Why can't he walk to the play yard by himself?" are common questions and demonstrate that children are paying attention to their environment and noticing, but not condemning, differences. Straightforward answers that do not reveal your own sense of frustration for the situation of a child with a disability is the best way to respond.

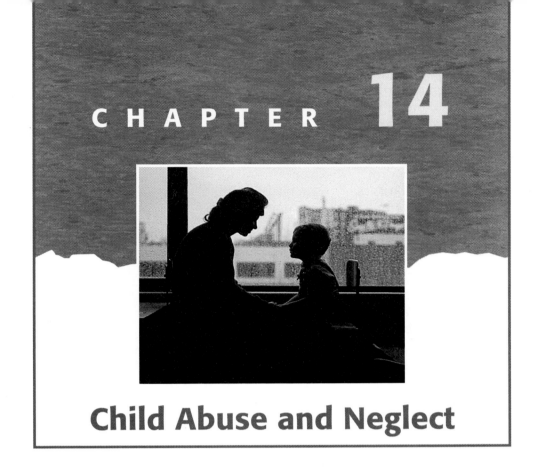

CHAPTER 14

Child Abuse and Neglect

Child abuse and neglect are tragic problems that cause suffering and fear for thousands of children. Child abuse is defined as physical injury, emotional mistreatment, neglect, or sexual abuse that is willfully inflicted on a child. Many children die each year from injuries received by abusive adults. Many more survive years of these abuses and suffer permanent damage physically, developmentally, and psychologically. An abused child often has low self-esteem and difficulty relating to others.

Child abuse and neglect occur at all levels of society and in all cultures. It is a very old problem that was quietly tolerated by society until recently. Fortunately, significant public and professional attention has forced society to no longer ignore a problem that jeopardizes the health and future of so many children.

Child care providers are trusted figures to young children. Their regular interaction with a small group of children allows them to observe closely a child's conduct and appearance and notice clues that might point towards a risk to the child's health and safety at home or elsewhere.

Today, children have a variety of exposures to adult authority figures, such as teachers, child care providers, parents, other relatives, parents' significant others, and teenage baby sitters. Children need to feel safe in the company of every adult who cares for them.

Physical Abuse

Physical abuse is a willful act of cruelty or violence against a child that results in an injury. It is often the result of unjustified or severe punishment and can occur when the adult is angry or frustrated and becomes violent towards the child with behaviors such as hitting, shaking, biting, throwing the child, or twisting a limb. Some abusive acts, such as burning or beating with a belt, are deliberate and premeditated. Often, physical abuse is a chronic situation. Frequent unexplained or poorly explained injuries or an injury that is unusual for the child's age, such as a fracture in an infant, should raise concern. Also of concern are injuries whose description does not seem plausible in light of the diagnosis from a health care provider.

What to Look For

The child's appearance:

- Head injuries are the most commonly cause of death from child abuse. Neurologic damage to the brain from a blow or from shaking can sometimes go undetected until pronounced symptoms develop, especially if there are no obvious signs of damage to the head or face.

- Scald burns are the most commonly inflicted burn injury. Some scalds result from hot liquids being thrown. Normally children withdraw immediately from pain, so that a well-defined margin on a burn like a mark around the ankle or wrist from the level of hot water, is suspicious. Immersion burns look like a glove on the hand or a sock on the foot. Pattern or branding burns are the shape of the item used, such as a cigarette or an iron, or round, such as a doughnut shape on the buttock from the burner of an electric stove.

- Burns from rope appear around the wrists or ankles if the child has been tied up.

- Bruises or welts can be located on hidden or visible areas of the body. Bruises on the buttocks, back, face, genitals, or paired small bruises from forceful pinching are all common.

- Broken bone injuries, especially those that occur more than once or those in which the description of how it happened does not coincide with the appearance of the injury

- Lacerations, especially on the face from a hand, a foot, or from the impact of a heavy object

- Bite marks appear as doughnut-shaped or double-horseshoe–shaped and may be discolored from bruising. In some bite marks, the tooth impressions help identify the biter, if they are shown to a health care provider promptly.

- Injuries in the mouth of an infant might indicate excessively forceful feeding.

The child's behavior:

- Becomes apprehensive when other children cry

- Appears afraid and hesitant to go with the abusive adult

- Is not trusting of physical contact with adults in the child care center

- Shows extremes of behavior from aggressiveness to isolation

- Might tell the child care provider what happened

Shaken Baby Syndrome

A severe degree of head injury can be inflicted on an infant who is roughly or violently shaken. Termed "shaken baby syndrome" or "shaken infant syndrome," it almost always occurs when a parent or other care giver shakes a crying baby in frustration to either punish or quiet the child. In most cases, it is the result of the adult losing self-control.

The infant's body proportions are very different from the adult's. Most significantly, the infant's head is oversized in comparison to the rest of the body and the neck muscles are not strong enough to support the head during rough handling. Shaking an infant causes the head to flop back and forth and the brain to bruise from banging against the skull wall.

This forceful shaking can result in bleeding, swelling and pressure in the brain, damage to the eyes, injuries to the neck and spine, and sometimes death. Often there are no outward signs of trauma to the body. The child who survives this injury can be left with a seizure disorder, severe visual impairment, some degree of paralysis, or mental retardation. Incidents of less violent shaking often leave the child with learning disabilities.

In rare instances, these injuries result accidentally from a parent or other adult tossing the infant in the air as an act of affection or play or from jogging with an infant in a backpack.

To prevent the devastating effects of shaken baby syndrome:

- Never shake an infant either in play or in anger.
- Call someone to stay with the infant or place the infant in a safe location, such as in the crib, and walk away if you feel out of control.
- Seek help from your local child abuse hotline for yourself or other care giver whose anger towards an infant causes you concern.

Emotional Abuse

Emotional abuse is continual verbal degradation and insults that cause the child to feel worthless and empty. It can damage the child intellectually, behaviorally, and psychologically. A parent's distorted view of parenting, harsh or inconsistent reactions to family life events, and verbal violence can create emotional problems that continue to affect the child later in life. Often emotional abuse accompanies physical abuse. Domestic violence witnessed by a child is also considered to be emotional abuse. If the child is repeatedly degraded for a long enough period of time, the child will begin to believe that what is communicated by the abuser is true. Unfortunately, emotional abuse is very difficult to prove.

What to Look For

The child's appearance:

- Signs of physical abuse
- Failure to thrive, described as abnormally low weight in conjunction with abnormally slow development for no apparent medical reason

The child's behavior:

- Lags behind in intellectual, physical, and emotional development
- Seems withdrawn and depressed
- Fluctuates emotionally between being unusually compliant and passive to being extremely aggressive, demanding, or violent
- Shows unusual adaptive behavior, such as being inappropriately adult (for instance, parenting other children) or inappropriately infantile (for example, thumb sucking, frequent rocking, and urinary incontinence)
- Is considered a behavior problem, showing self-destructive behavior and might eventually attempt suicide
- Makes statements such as, "Daddy says I'm a very bad boy."

Sexual Abuse

Sexual abuse consists of inappropriate physical contact with a child. This covers a wide range of crimes from fondling and indecent exposure to violent activities such as rape. Most cases of sexual abuse are recurrent and the child knows the sexual offender. The child might be sworn to secrecy by an abuser who has bribed the child or threatened violence or death of the child or another loved one if the child tells anyone.

What to Look For

The child's appearance:

- Irritation, pain, bruises, or bleeding in the genital area
- Discharge from the vagina or penis that could be from a sexually transmitted disease
- Stained or bloody underwear

The child's behavior:

- Has poor relationships with peers and withdraws from social activities
- Engages in abnormal fantasy or infantile behavior
- Has recurrent nightmares that might be shared with child care staff
- Has a greater conversational knowledge of sexual matters than is appropriate for his or her age
- Has inappropriate and excessive curiosity about sexual matters or private body parts of others
- Shows fear or hesitancy about going with a particular person
- Exhibits regressive behavior (in school-aged children), such as thumb sucking, crying excessively, and withdrawing into a fantasy world
- Engages in other behaviors (in school-aged children), including aggressive or disruptive acting out, running away, delinquent activities, and failing in school work
- Might report incidents indirectly, such as, " I know someone who . . ." or " What would you do if . . . ?"
- Has problems with pants-wetting and fecal soiling

Neglect

A chronically neglected child suffers from a lack of care and protection, which can have an injurious effect on physical and emotional health. These children suffer from inadequate nutrition, clothing, shelter, personal and household hygiene, and medical care. Too often they lack proper supervision. They also lack consistent contact with nurturing and supportive adults outside of the child care setting. Children who are neglected in these ways are vulnerable to disease, injury, and a variety of social problems.

What to Look For

The child's appearance:

- Has untreated medical problems and rarely sees a health care provider or a dentist for well-child care

- Looks unkempt, is inadequately dressed—especially in cold weather, looks and smells dirty, and has chronic mouth odor

- Conversation reveals that the child is often alone, cared for by another child, or engages in activities that are dangerous or inappropriate for his or her age

- Conversation causes you to suspect that home is unsanitary or lacks adequate heating or plumbing

The child's behavior:

- Little experience with rules and limit-setting

- Behavior might appear delinquent compared with behavior of other children in the center or school

- Frequent use of foul language, which can indicate that the adults or older children to whom the child is exposed outside of the child care center speak inappropriately

- Frequent complaints of hunger and sneaking of food

- Often tired and lacks enthusiasm

- Has a poor attendance record with unexplained absences

How to Help

All adults need to be aware of the devastation that abuse in any form brings upon a child and must be willing to get involved. Child care providers and teachers are, in many states, defined as professionals who are required by law to report suspected child abuse to the state's protective services.

Some child care providers worry about hurting a trusted relationship with a young child by breaking confidentiality. It is important to report suspected abuse when you first become suspicious, because abuse is more often a pattern than a one-time incident and is likely to continue or even intensify. It is important that you not tell the child that you will keep this shared information a secret, but rather let the child know that you can help. You are a key person in recognizing the signs of child abuse and getting the system working to rescue a child from an abusive situation or find services and support to help a dysfunctional family heal. For more information about how to help a child when abuse is suspected, call the National Child Abuse Hotline at 1-800-422-4453.

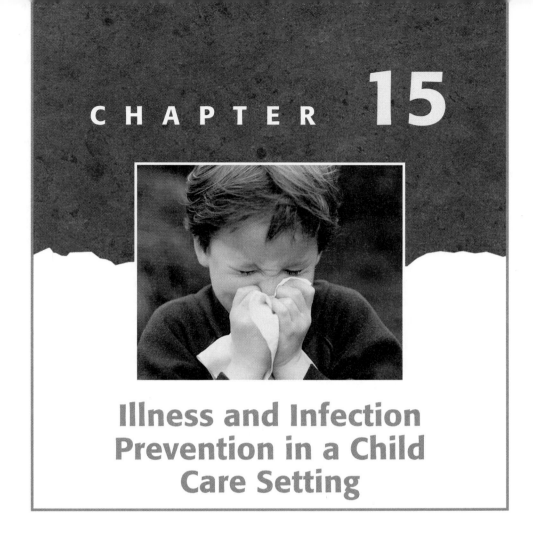

CHAPTER 15

Illness and Infection Prevention in a Child Care Setting

Some children are the picture of health no matter what the season. Other children seem to pick up every illness to which they are exposed. On the average, toddlers and preschoolers experience six to eight episodes of illness each year. This frequency decreases to about three episodes each year by the time a child is 6 years old. Fortunately, the incidence of many of the serious and life-threatening childhood illnesses has been dramatically reduced by vaccines and antibiotics. Today in the United States common illnesses are generally mild compared to those of past generations.

What Causes Illness
Viruses

Infections caused by viruses include illnesses such as chicken pox, colds, croup, some pneumonias, and the gastrointestinal upsets of vomiting and diarrhea. Symptoms that accompany viral infections such as cough, congestion, and fever can be treated to make the child feel more comfortable. Pharmaceutical companies are working to develop medications to treat viral infections, but for now there are no medications available. Antibiotics have no effect on viruses. Most illness caused by viruses subside with time.

The viruses that cause the common cold, as well as many of the common upper respiratory infections, enter through the eyes, nose, and mouth. They are spread from one person to another as airborne particles from a cough or a sneeze or by direct contact. If children sneeze into their hands and then pick up toys or touch a door knob without first washing their hands, they will contaminate these items with the virus.

Bacteria

Bacterial infections, which include illnesses such as ear infections, strep throat, scarlet fever, impetigo, and some pneumonias, must be treated by prescription antibiotics to ensure prompt and complete recovery. To help prevent an infection from recurring, it is important for a child taking an antibiotic to complete the entire course of medicine.

Fungi

Fungal infections include such conditions as ringworm, athlete's foot, and thrush; they are usually not serious. There are several medications for fungal infections. Antibiotics are not prescribed to treat fungal infections and, in some instances, can worsen the condition.

Intestinal Parasites

Intestinal parasitic infections such as pinworms and giardia are common and are caused by worms and protozoa. They are transmitted by ingestion and need to be treated with a prescription medication specifically for the parasite.

How Illness Is Spread

Microorganisms that cause illness enter the body in one of these four ways:

Direct contact or touching, as with the impetigo bacteria, the herpesvirus, and the thrush fungus

Ingestion, as with the pinworm parasite and the hepatitis A virus

Airborne transmission of microorganisms through the eyes, nose, or mouth, as with the common cold, influenza, and chicken pox viruses or the strep throat bacteria

Blood to blood contact, as with the HIV virus.

Preventing Infection in a Child Care Setting

Most young children attend either a nursery school or a child care setting in their preschool years. Spending many hours each day inside and in close contact with several other youngsters invites the spread of illness. To decrease the incidence of illness among children, care givers must consistently practice good hygiene and encourage children to follow their example. Do all the staff members in your center use the following good hygiene rules?

1. **Wash hands frequently.** This is the single most important measure you can take to prevent the spread of illness and infection.

   How to wash hands:

   - Use liquid soap and warm water to scrub hands vigorously for 15 to 30 seconds. The friction created by rubbing hands together contributes as much to the cleaning as the soap and water does. Also wash the backs of the hands and under the fingernails.

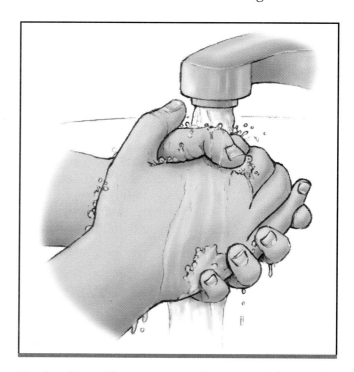

Handwashing with warm soap and water can help stop the spread of disease.

   - Rinse clean hands with warm running water and dry them with a clean paper towel. Then use the towel to turn off the water faucet and discard the towel.

- Fingernails should be kept short and scrubbed with a nail brush. Organisms collect easily under long fingernails.

When to wash hands:

- Before eating or preparing foods
- After toileting, helping a child with toileting, or diapering
- After touching any body fluid such as saliva, nasal discharge, blood, tears, stool, or urine, and after removing disposable gloves

When to have children wash their hands:

- After toileting. Young children need to be taught, reminded, and supervised. Infants and toddlers who wear diapers should have their hands washed after diaper changes if they touch their diaper area.
- After playing outside
- Before participating in a cooking project
- Before meal and snack times
- Before playing with play dough

2. **Disinfect all washable surfaces.** Use a commercial disinfectant or a sanitizing solution of bleach and water. The solution should be made of one part bleach to ten parts water and must be made fresh daily. It is inexpensive and extremely effective in killing microorganisms. Spray it on all washable surfaces and allow it to air dry. The following areas should be disinfected daily:

- Sinks
- Toilets
- Potty seats
- Diaper changing tables
- Table tops
- Door knobs

  Mouthed toys should be washed daily, rinsed with the sanitizing solution, rinsed with water, and allowed to air dry.

  Vomit, diarrhea, and blood should be wiped up with gloved hands, and the surface should be disinfected. Soiled clothing and bedding should be placed in a plastic bag and sent home with the child.

3. **Use disposable gloves.** Disposable nonporous gloves made from latex, rubber, nitrile, or other hypoallergenic materials act as a barrier between your skin and another person's body

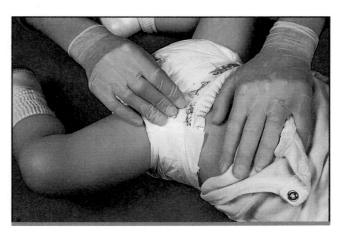

Changing a diaper

fluids, such as blood, diarrhea, urine, and vomit. Gloves should be worn when there is a chance of touching these fluids, because of the many organisms that can be present in these fluids and transmit disease. Gloves also protect a child with an open wound from contaminants on the child care provider's hands.

Disposable gloves should be available in each bathroom, in the diaper changing area, and in the first aid kit. Wash hands thoroughly with soap and water after removing disposable gloves. Throw the gloves away after one use.

4. **Practice good hygiene and encourage the children to follow your example.**

- Tie long hair back.
- Do not share personal items, such as combs, brushes, hats, toothbrushes, cups, and drinking straws.
- Keep fingernails clean and trimmed.
- Do not bite fingernails, rub eyes, or otherwise touch the face without washing hands first. Touching the face and mouth can introduce germs that cause colds and other illnesses. Turn your head toward the floor or cover your mouth when coughing and sneezing.
- Use disposable tissues for coughing, sneezing, and wiping a nose. Dispose of soiled tissues promptly.
- Spend part of every day outside with the children, weather permitting.
- Leave the doors and windows open while the children are outside, weather permitting, so that fresh air can circulate through the building.

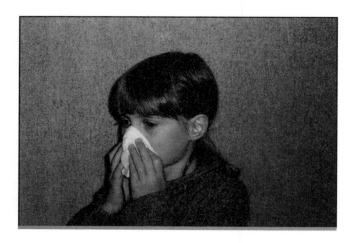

- Child care staff, parents, and visitors should not smoke in the child care center.
- Practice good hygiene routinely, not just when a child is ill.

5. **Maintain clean inside and outside play areas.**

- Drain wading pools daily and as needed. Drain, clean, and disinfect water tables daily and allow them to air dry. Clean and disinfect water toys.
- Cover outside sandboxes. If left uncovered, sandboxes can become litter boxes for cats and other animals. The ingestion of microscopic particles of infected animal waste can cause illness.
- Put rubber pants over diapers, even disposable diapers, when taking a young child into a wading pool.
- Lawn sprinklers are more hygienic than wading pools for water play in the summer.

6. **Handle and prepare foods properly.**

- Wash hands before handling food. Be aware of what you touch during preparation and rewash hands as necessary.
- Tie hair back, or wear a hair net.
- Do not handle food when you are ill.

- Avoid changing diapers if you are a food preparer. In a home child care setting, where there is only one provider, good hand washing technique is essential.
- Keep the diaper-changing area separate from the food area.
- Do not taste the food with a utensil that is used to cook and stir.
- Use separate surfaces and utensils when preparing meat.
- Wash all dishes and eating utensils in an automatic dishwasher with the booster thermostat set to 170°F. If a dishwasher is unavailable, wash dishes and utensils with hot water and soap, rinse in a sanitizing solution of bleach (ten parts water to one part bleach), rinse again with clear water, and allow to air dry. If your center does not have proper cleaning facilities, disposable dishes and utensils must be used and then discarded.

7. **Take special precautions with infants.**

- Wash mouthed toys daily with hot water and soap, rinse in a sanitizing solution of bleach (ten parts water to one part bleach), rinse again with clear water, and allow to air dry.
- Rinse a pacifier or a toy that was dropped on the floor before handing it back to an infant.
- Wear a disposable or cloth gown when holding an infant under 6 months of age.
- Use a separate gown for each infant.

Many states have specific written requirements concerning infection control in a child care center. In addition, many child care centers have their own written guidelines developed or approved by a health care consultant. Your center's staff should know the state guidelines.

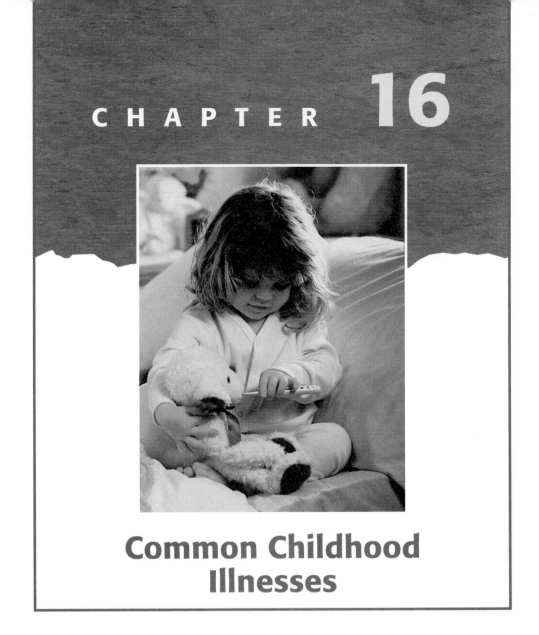

CHAPTER 16

Common Childhood Illnesses

Many of the bouts of illness that children experience in their early years are caused by the "garden variety" of viruses and are destroyed by the child's immune system in a matter of days. Some viral illnesses are more persistent and the child takes longer to bounce back. A sick child should be monitored by a parent or care giver to be sure that the child stays on the road to recovery or, if a complication develops, care is sought immediately.

Colds, diarrhea, fever, and vomiting are four common ailments that are actually symptoms or a collection of symptoms of an infection. Usually, these infections are caused by viruses, and less often by bacteria. These common ailments recur a number of times in young children. They occur year round but more often during the fall and winter months when colder temperatures and inclement weather keep windows closed and people closely together. With children coughing or simply breathing their germs around the enclosed space of a child care center or home care setting, viral infections spread easily. Because the breeze blowing through the building really does clear the air by diluting the concentration of infective organisms in it, leaving doors or windows open for a few minutes when the children are outdoors is of benefit to everyone.

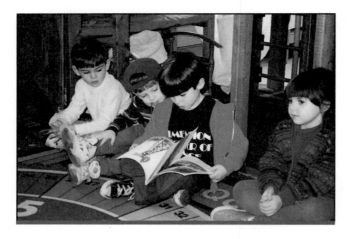

Colds

By far the most common ailment of young children is the common cold, which is caused by viruses and must run its course. Symptoms, including a runny or stuffy nose, sore throat, and cough, can last from 4 days to 2 weeks. A child might also have a fever during a cold, particularly at the beginning, as well as a headache and temporarily decreased hearing and appetite. "Not acting like herself" is often the best indicator of how sick the child feels. Most colds are not serious. The chief problem for child care providers and parents is keeping the child happy and the symptoms under control.

What to Do

1. Use over-the-counter decongestants and cough medicines as recommended by the child's health care provider.

2. Use a cool-mist vaporizer in the child care setting and at home in the child's bedroom at night. This reduces congestion by keeping mucus thin and allowing it to drain. The vaporizer must be cleaned daily with soap and water, then rinsed with a solution of one part bleach to ten parts water. Cool mist is as effective as hot steam and is much safer near young children.

3. Parents can break up congestion in a stuffy nose with either salt water or plain water nose drops. Salt water nose drops are made by mixing ¼ teaspoon table salt in ½ cup (4 ounces) of water. Use an eye dropper, available in the drug store, to instill a few drops in each nostril while the child lies on the back. This loosens the dry mucus and allows it to run out of the nose or be suctioned away with a nasal aspirator and can be done several times per day.

4. Use a nasal aspirator (suction bulb) for infants. To use, press the bulb flat and hold the tip at the opening or just inside the nostril; release and remove. This is especially helpful before meals and at bedtime and a few minutes after instilling salt water or plain water nose drops.

5. The parent should call the child's health care provider if the child develops a fever, complains of pain in the ear or elsewhere, the nasal drainage becomes yellow or green, or the eyes develop a discharge or become crusty.

Trying to teach toddlers or preschoolers to blow their nose can be tricky. For some children, this ability develops eventually but is hard to understand before the child is ready for it. If too young, it is likely that the child will suck in rather than blow out, which only leads to further mucus congestion. For the child ready to learn to blow the nose, try suggesting that the child think of blowing out birthday candles through the nose. This helps to start the purposeful exhalation necessary for success.

Diarrhea

When a child has diarrhea, the bowel movements, or stools, are loose (either mushy or very watery) and more frequent than is normal for the child. Sometimes diarrhea is accompanied by vomiting, stomach pain, or fever. Common causes are viral illness, antibiotic treatment (which upsets the balance of normal bacteria in the intestines), or a dietary cause (either a particular food or the quantity of a food). Less commonly, certain illnesses or bacterial or parasitic infections cause diarrhea. See Common Childhood Illnesses chart, *Infectious Diarrhea.*

A young child with infectious diarrhea or diarrhea that cannot be contained should be kept at home until the necessary treatment is completed and negative results are obtained on stool cultures. Treating diarrhea involves giving the bowel a rest while giving the child enough fluid to replace what is lost in the stools. Diarrhea is especially worrisome in infants, because a very small body can become dehydrated easily. See *Dehydration,* Chapter 12. Most diarrhea, however, resolves without treatment within a few days.

What to Do

1. **Keep the fluid intake high.** During an acute episode of diarrhea, do not give solid food, but encourage small sips of clear fluids (fluids you can see through). Big gulps can cause another burst of diarrhea. Good choices for clear fluids are a pediatric electrolyte solution available in grocery and drug stores, a diluted sports drink, canned fruit drinks mixed with an equal amount of water, or gelatin water made with twice as much water as the instructions state. Clear fluids alone should not be given for more than 24 hours.

   For infants: If breastfeeding, continue and offer a pediatric electrolyte solution between feedings. If formula feeding, temporarily discontinue formula and give the pediatric electrolyte solution. A good substitute, if this solution is not available, is gelatin water made with twice as much water. Clear fluids alone should not be given for more than 24 hours.

2. **Provide good skin care.** Change diapers immediately and wash and dry the skin well after each diarrhea episode. Petroleum jelly creates a moisture barrier for the skin. Skin irritation caused by diarrhea may be so uncomfortable that even toilet-trained children complain of a burning sensation of the skin around the anus. Wash your hands well after every diaper change or toileting assistance because diarrhea can be contagious.

3. **Slowly return to a regular diet.** Once the diarrhea begins to improve, slowly begin to offer foods that bind and slow the passage of stool through the intestines, such as bananas, applesauce, white toast without butter or margarine, crackers, rice cakes, dry cereals, noodles, rice, and other low-fat, bland foods. Continue to encourage fluids. Temporarily avoid milk products and other fruits. As the child improves further, slowly return to the regular diet. Return milk, cheese, and ice cream to the diet last because they are difficult to digest.

   For infants: Offer applesauce, bananas, carrots, and rice cereal to infants on solid food. Slowly return to full-strength formula or offer a soy formula for several days, because it is more easily digested than a milk formula.

The child's health care provider might have a preferred regimen for diarrhea management.

When Diarrhea Becomes Worrisome

The parent should call the child's health care provider if:

- The child is an infant under 6 months of age.
- The child is unable to drink.
- The child shows any signs of dehydration, such as dry lips and mouth, listlessness, no tears when crying, a dry diaper for several hours, or infrequent, small amounts of deep gold urine.
- The child complains of severe abdominal pain.
- There is blood, pus, or mucus in the stool.
- Diarrhea has not improved at all in 24 hours.
- Mild or moderate diarrhea persists longer than 1 week, indicating that a stool culture might be necessary.
- The child's diarrhea appears to be caused by an antibiotic medicine.

DO NOT

- offer apple juice, because it aggravates diarrhea in some children.
- offer carbonated beverages or powdered drink mixes.

Fever

A fever is an elevated temperature. Fevers are very common in young children. The arrival of a fever triggers a period of discomfort and illness for the child and concern for the parents. A fever is not an illness; it is a symptom of an illness. It is not harmful and, in fact, is beneficial in fighting an illness. However, a prolonged fever can be of concern when the illness responsible for it is not diagnosed and treated.

Why does a child get a fever? When the body's defense system, known as the immune system, finds an invading organism, such as a bacteria or a virus, certain "fighter" blood cells surround the invader to destroy it. This triggers a message to the brain to "turn up the heat." The higher body temperature created by the fever helps the fighter cells because they work more effectively at temperatures above normal. A fever is worrisome in a child under the age of 6 months (and especially under 3 months), because a young infant cannot fight infection as easily as older children and can more easily become dehydrated.

The normal oral temperature reading is 98.6°F. During an illness, it is not unusual for a young child's fever to run as high as 105°F. A temperature can be measured orally, rectally, or under the arm (axillary) with a standard glass or digital thermometer or in the ear with a small probe that measures the infrared heat produced in the eardrum and surrounding tissue.

Readings vary depending on where the temperature is taken. The method you use depends on the age of the child. Taking the temperature rectally gives the most accurate reading; however, it is unnecessarily intrusive to an older child. A rectal temperature reading registers one degree higher than an oral temperature reading. An axillary temperature reading registers one degree lower than an oral reading.

A glass thermometer can take up to 1 minute to register rectally, 3 minutes to register orally, and 10 minutes to register under the arm. Some glass thermometers are designed for oral use and others for rectal use. A digital thermometer can be used to take either an oral, rectal, or axillary temperature and takes only 1 minute to register. An ear probe heat sensor takes only seconds to register and the reading is comparable to an oral temperature reading.

Taking an oral temperature is not recommended for children age 4 and under because the skill of holding the thermometer under the tongue with the mouth closed while breathing through the nose is beyond their understanding and capability. Avoid giving a cold drink if taking an oral temperature because it will make the reading inaccurate.

What to Do

The fever remains for as long as the immune system is fighting the invading organism. Since a fever is not an illness in itself, it is not possible to speed up the process or "cure" the fever. A moderate fever (99°F to 102°F) can promote the body's infection-fighting system without the child's discomfort and the parental worry that a fever above 102°F causes.

1. Separate the child from other children and notify the child's parent, because a fever is often associated with a contagious illness. The child should remain at home until fever-free for 24 hours or, if necessary, until examined by a health care provider.

2. Encourage sips of clear fluids (fluids you can see through), such as water, tea, "flat" ginger ale, finely crushed ice, popsicles, and gelatin. Apple juice is a clear fluid but it can cause diarrhea in some children and should be avoided.

3. Give acetaminophen if the fever is above 101°F. Give the recommended dosage prescribed by the child's health care provider. Know your center's policy regarding the administration of medication. A parent might find it helpful to have children's acetaminophen suppositories on hand. They are an easy way to get fever-reducing medicine into a child who is also nauseated, is vomiting, or is too ill to swallow liquid or pills. They can be purchased over-the-counter but are kept under refrigeration, so you must ask for them.

4. Dress the child as lightly as possible, but do not allow the child to shiver. Shivering closes the skin pores and can increase the body temperature. The child feels alternately hot and cold as the fever goes up and down.

5. Sponge bathe a child if the fever is over 103°F. Rub the skin briskly using tepid water (75°F to 85°F) and a face cloth. Keep the water warm enough so that the child does not shiver. Wet the head because almost half of the body's heat loss is through the head. As the water evaporates, cooling of the body occurs.

Recommended Methods for Taking Child's Temperature by Age

Age of Child	Method			
	Rectal	Axillary	Oral	Auricular
1 year and younger	●	●		●
2 years		●		●
3 years		●		●
4 years		●		●
5 years and older			●	●

Axillary = under the arm
Auricular = in the ear (with a special probe)

Reye's syndrome is an uncommon disease that affects all organs of the body, especially the liver and brain. It strikes quickly and is most likely to occur during the recovery period after a viral illness, such as influenza, upper respiratory infections, and chicken pox. It is not contagious. Symptoms include unexpected and continuous vomiting, confusion and delirium, combativeness and other irrational behavior, drowsiness, convulsion, and coma. The body temperature usually remains normal. A child with Reye's syndrome requires hospitalization for treatment. Fortunately, the sudden and severe onset of symptoms almost guarantees that the child's health care provider will be called promptly.

Although there is no known cause for the disease, some studies suggest that there is a link between the development of Reye's syndrome and the use of aspirin for viral illnesses. The U.S. Surgeon General, the Food and Drug Administration, and the Centers for Disease Control now recommend that children not be given aspirin (also called salicylate) and products that contain aspirin for fever unless specifically recommended by a health care provider. Many manufacturers of aspirin voluntarily label their products with this warning, and many pharmacies place warnings beside their aspirin products. Reye's syndrome has also developed in children who were not taking aspirin for their illnesses.

DO NOT

- give aspirin or any product containing salicylate to a child with a fever unless a health care provider tells you to do so.
- sponge bathe with cold water or put the child in a tub of cold water. It will make the child shiver.
- use rubbing alcohol on the skin to reduce a fever. It feels cold enough to cause shivering, is absorbed by the skin, and is poisonous to the central nervous system.
- force foods into a child with a fever. When a child has a fever, drinking is important; eating is not.
- use these instructions to treat a child with an extremely high temperature from heat stroke.

Vomiting

Nausea and vomiting are common symptoms of a stomach virus and should last no longer than 24 hours. A slight fever or diarrhea might accompany the nausea and vomiting. The obvious worry about vomiting is that it can lead to dehydration. A young child who is vomiting should be removed from child care and kept home until the child feels better.

What to Do

1. Give nothing to eat or drink until 1 hour has passed since the child last vomited.

2. After 1 hour has passed, offer one tablespoon of water or ice chips every 15 to 20 minutes to keep the child adequately hydrated. Big gulps will likely result in more vomiting. Offer a wet face cloth for the child to suck on to keep the mouth and lips moist. If the child begins to vomit again, allow the stomach to rest for another 30 minutes to 1 hour and then start over. If the child tolerates small sips of water for 1 hour, offer sips of other clear fluids, such as tea, "flat" ginger ale or cola (shaken until all bubbles are gone), a diluted sports drink, a pediatric electrolyte solution (available in grocery and drug stores), gelatin water made with twice as much water, canned fruit drinks mixed with equal parts of water, or popsicles.

3. Wait several hours before offering food. Begin with foods that are easily tolerated, such as rice

The parent should call the child's health care provider if:

- The child is an infant under 6 months of age.
- The child is unable to keep any fluid in the stomach for several hours.
- The child shows any signs of dehydration, such as dry lips and mouth, listlessness, no tears when crying, a dry diaper for several hours, or infrequent, small amounts of deep gold urine.
- The child complains of severe stomach or abdominal pain.
- Vomiting is forceful and projectile.
- There is blood in the vomit.

cakes, dry cereal, dry toast, and crackers. Avoid offering solids and clear liquids together, because they might cause a return of nausea or vomiting.

For infants:
Offer applesauce, bananas, and rice cereal. The child should be back on a regular diet within 1 to 2 days after the vomiting.

DO NOT

- **stop breast-feeding unless instructed to do so by your child's health care provider.**

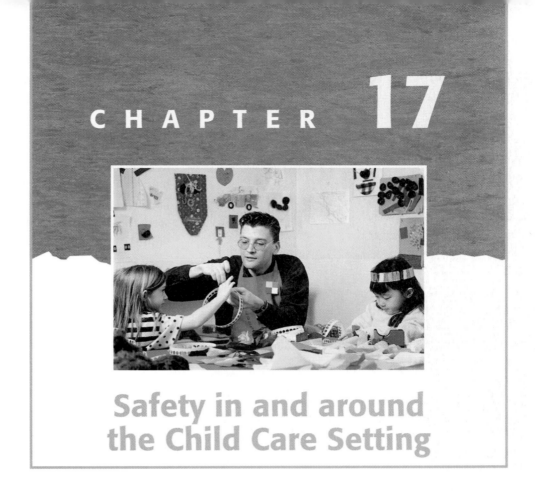

CHAPTER 17

Safety in and around the Child Care Setting

Young children are driven by nature to learn about their environment by exploring and by using their senses of taste and touch. Because they cannot make judgments about their own health and safety, this drive puts them at risk for injuries, such as burns, falls, choking, drowning, and poisoning.

A child care provider's understanding of growth and development is invaluable in creating a hazard-free environment full of safe and age-appropriate items. It is essential to identify and remove all potential dangers. Safety is an even greater challenge in family child care settings and family homes, because children are likely to be of different ages and at different developmental stages there. Creative spacing of play areas and thoughtful storage of toys may be required.

As children grow, be aware that hazards change because of their advancing capabilities. Remember that a mobile child's possibilities for adventure—both horizontal and vertical—are endless.

Read about preventing burn injuries and fires in Chapter 6. Read about preventing poisonings in Chapter 9.

Indoor Safety

Spend some time in each room of the child care center or home examining it for safety hazards that might injure a child.

Basement (see Garage, Basement, and Laundry Area)

Common Injuries Related to Child's Developmental Level

Developmental Characteristics	Potential Injuries
Infant - Age 0 to 1 year	
Increasing mobility	Burns
Uses mouth to explore objects	Choking
Reaches for and pulls objects	Drowning
Unaware of dangers	Falls
Cannot understand "no"	
Toddler - Age 1 to 2½ years	
Masters walking, running, climbing	Burns
Explores almost everything with mouth	Choking
Begins to imitate behaviors	Drowning
Investigates everything within reach	Falls
Curious about all never-before-seen items	Pedestrian injuries
Unaware of most dangers	Poisoning
Impulsive	Suffocation
Preschooler- Age 2½ to 5 years	
Mobility leads to increased independence	Burns
	Choking
Learns to ride tricycle	Drowning
Unaware of many dangers	Falls
Might favor real, rather than toy, tools, gadgets, appliances	Pedestrian injuries
Fascinated with fire	Poisoning
Imitates adult behavior	
School-aged - Age 5 years and up	
Needs to be independent	Bicycle injuries
Needs to be like peers	Burns
Needs to be with peers	Falls
Needs increased physical activity	Pedestrian injuries
Dangers do not always seem real	
Increased independence can mean less closely supervised	Firearm injuries

Bathroom

- Keep the toilet lid down. Do not use continuous blue or bleach-containing bowl cleaners.
- Keep the bathroom door closed to keep very young children out entirely.
- Use a rubber mat or nonskid decals in the bathtub and shower stall.
- Cover the bath tub faucet with a plastic sponge cover to prevent injury.
- Set the temperature of the hot water heater not to exceed 110°F. See more about preventing burn injuries in the bathroom in *Preventing Burn Injuries* in Chapter 6.
- Keep electrical bathroom appliances, such as hair blow dryers, away from water.
- Lock the bathroom medicine cabinet. Do not store medicines or chemicals underneath the bathroom sink.

Bedroom

- Use a standard-size crib, which has a mattress that fits snugly. If two fingers can fit between the mattress and crib, the mattress is too small. See more about crib safety in *Infant Equipment Safety*.
- Use a changing table with a safety strap. Never leave a baby unattended on a changing table, even when strapped.
- To prevent falls, change clothes and diapers of active infants and toddlers on the floor rather than on a table.
- At bedtime, be sure that toys are well out of the path between the bed and the bedroom door.
- Do not place any furniture on which a child might climb under a bedroom window.
- Open double-hung windows from the top down if above the first floor. This allows for the same amount of breeze but keeps the glass window at the child's level to prevents falls. Some states and private agencies provide financial support for obtaining child-safety screens for windows. Check with your local Public Health Department.
- Do not let a child sit on a windowsill.
- Use a bed side guard when a young child is first moved from a crib to a bed.
- Use a sturdy bed side guard for a top bunk and do not allow young children to play or sleep on the top bunk.

Garage, Basement, and Laundry Area

- Children should be kept out of these areas if hazardous chemicals and equipment are stored without child safety in mind.

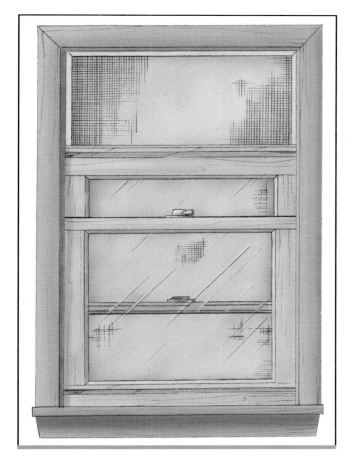

Open double-hung windows from the top.

- Install a hook and eye latch above the child's reach on the entrance door to these areas.
- Keep chemicals stored in these areas in their original containers. Place them on high shelves or, preferably, in a locked cabinet. Purchase corrosive chemicals, such as drain cleaners, in one-use quantities whenever possible.
- Avoid interruption when using a poisonous product. If you must leave your work area, put the chemical safely away or carry it with you.
- Unplug appliances, such as an iron or power tools, and keep them as well as garden tools out of reach.
- Store ropes and cords out of children's reach.
- Keep the washer and dryer doors closed.
- Lock a freezer or extra refrigerator kept in any of these areas.

Kitchen

- Post emergency telephone numbers next to your kitchen phone and next to every other phone.

- Cook on back burners whenever possible to prevent children from touching hot elements or flame. See more about preventing burn injuries in the kitchen in *Preventing Burn Injuries* in Chapter 6.
- Do not store household cleaning products alongside food. The differences between them might not be apparent to a young child.
- Keep products in their original, labeled containers. Do not reuse empty containers, such as juice bottles, paper cups, or empty food containers.
- Use plastic latches or other safety latches on kitchen cupboards and drawers that contain dangerous items, such as knives and heavy appliances or cookware. Poisons should not be stored behind plastic safety latches. Designate one lower cupboard away from the stove as the child's, and stock it with lightweight plastic items so that the child can be safely occupied when you are working in the kitchen.
- Keep heavy objects and appliances with cords such as blenders, food processors, or small TVs far enough away from the edge of the countertop or table so that a young child cannot reach them.
- Do not allow a child to play at your feet while you are cooking. There is too great a risk for injury to both of you from a burn, fall, or cut.
- To prevent falls, wipe up spills immediately and limit the use of floor wax or polish.
- Position a high chair away from busy areas so that a child cannot reach the stove, countertop, or electric or phone cords. See more about high chairs in *Infant Equipment Safety* in this chapter.
- Do not allow children to chew on styrofoam cups and food containers. Particles can be inhaled causing respiratory irritation.

Laundry Area (see *Garage, Basement, and Laundry Area*)

Living Area

- Install smoke detectors. Check the batteries in the spring and fall when you change your clocks. See more about preventing burn injuries in the living area in *Preventing Burn Injuries* in Chapter 6.
- Anchor tall and unsteady bookcases to the walls.

- Rearrange furniture if sharp corners on tables protrude into areas of heavy traffic.

- Do not leave such dangerous items as hot beverages, scissors, or breakable pieces on a low table, such as a coffee table.

- Place decorative stickers at a child's eye level on large sliding glass doors to prevent injury from a child colliding with the glass.

Stairs

- Be cautious when using expandable doorway gates at stairwells. If you use an accordion-type gate with large diamond-shaped openings, be sure the gate has a safety rail along the top to eliminate the V-shaped openings where children can entrap their heads. Some children try to climb these gates. Safer gate models are tension gates made entirely of plastic or plastic mesh on a wooden frame, both of which snap closed in doorways. Use gates only for the doorway widths suggested by the manufacturer. Do not climb over a doorway gate yourself because children often mimic adults.

- Make stairs skid-proof with carpet or rubber mats. Place skid-proof padding under all small area rugs or hallway rugs.

- Repair or replace torn carpeting on the stairs because of the risk of tripping and falling.

- Check that handrails are secured to the wall.

- Keep the stairway area open and free of toys. Do not allow children to play near a stairway.

- Keep the stairway area well lit.

- Teach young children to descend stairs by crawling down backwards.

Inside or Outside the Building

- Test paint on the windows and window sills and on the exterior of the building for lead content. Call your Department of Public Health to learn about procedures to follow. Should de-leading be necessary, children must not be present. See *Lead Poisoning in Children.*

- Test your child care center or home for the presence of radon. Radon is a lung-cancer–causing radioactive gas that you cannot see, smell, or taste. It comes from the natural breakdown of uranium under the ground and gets into buildings through cracks in the basement or other foundations. There are many

ways to solve a radon problem in a building. Obtain a testing kit in your local hardware store or by contacting your state radon office. For more information, call the National Radon Hotline at 1-800-SOS-RADON.

Infant Equipment Safety

Young children are usually very active, whether they are on the floor or in one of the many pieces of equipment designed to meet their needs and yours. Because they cannot evaluate possible hazards, they can be injured in what seem to be safest places.

Standards and guidelines for juvenile equipment have been improved over the years by the U.S. Consumer Product Safety Commission. Check older hand-me-down or yard-sale–purchased equipment before using it, making certain that it conforms to current standards and guidelines.

Cribs

Current federal regulations require the following:

- Standard-size cribs must have mattresses that fit snugly. If two fingers can fit between the mattress and crib, the mattress is too small.

- Crib slats must be no more than $2\frac{3}{8}$ inches apart. This ensures that infants cannot slip through and become strangled or trapped. Do not use a crib with decorative openings in the end panels that would allow head or limb entrapment. Do not use a crib with a broken or missing slat.

- Corner posts must not stick up above the front and back panels by more than $\frac{1}{16}$ inch to prevent entanglement of clothing or cords.

- There must be no rough edges or metal hardware inside the crib.

- Locks on the side rails must not be accessible to a child, who might release them.

Your responsibility checklist includes:

- Make sure that your crib meets all of the above standards.

- Make sure that the metal mattress support hangers are secure on the head and foot board posts.

- Do not allow drapery or blind cords to hang near a crib. Do not string toys from rail to rail or across a crib. Both present a risk for strangulation.

Lead Poisoning in Children

The toxic effects of lead on the human body has caused the United States government to name it the country's number one environmental threat to children. Unlike many environmental health problems, lead is often found right at home in drinking water, household paint, house dust, and outdoor soil. Lead is especially damaging to children under age 6. The tragedy of lead poisoning is that there are few symptoms to warn a parent in the early stages. Often the poisoning is not diagnosed until there is some degree of irreparable brain damage, causing developmental delays, behavioral problems, and intellectual impairment. There is recent evidence that lead is toxic at blood levels once thought safe. Lower IQ scores, slower development, attention problems, and kidney and stomach problems have been observed in children with very low blood lead levels.

Infants and toddlers can come in contact with lead-contaminated dust and soil often, because they spend a lot of time on the floor or ground and often have their hands in their mouths. Most homes built before 1960 have some lead paint inside or on the exterior, which ends up in the air or the soil as the paint ages. Even more serious are the higher doses of the toxic metal that young children receive when they eat tiny chips of old leaded paint. Lead dust can be found in high concentration in home renovation projects, where lead paint is disturbed, and on windows, window sills, or older porch floors, where it is ground up by the simple friction of walking. Some older homes also have lead water pipes and lead-soldered copper pipes from which lead can leech into the water, especially into hot water. Some other sources of lead include: lead-glazed pottery and leaded crystal and china, food or drink cans soldered with lead, some brightly-colored imported painted toys, colored newsprint, and cigarettes. Screening children for lead is generally done between 1 and 2 years of age and earlier if the child's risk of exposure is higher than average.

The following recommendations will help you protect children from harmful lead exposure:

- Test exterior and interior paint in your home or child care center to determine if the paint contains lead. Take the necessary steps to remove it safely if it is present.

- Test the water in your home or center for lead. If there is lead in your water, it is likely caused by corrosion in your plumbing.

- Test the soil around your home for lead. If lead is present, plant grass or other ground cover around the house to make the soil less accessible to children.

- Keep children away from peeling or chipping paint on accessible surfaces, such as window sills.

- Provide a sand box with a wooden or plastic bottom and a lid for children to play in.

- Do not use unglazed pottery or leaded crystal or china or pottery meant for decorative use to serve food or drink.

- Do not let children play with or mouth brightly painted imported toys, colored newsprint, or old kitchen utensils with painted handles.

- Use crib bumper pads, mobiles, and crib gyms only until the child can push up onto hands and knees; then remove them.

- When the child can pull up to a standing position, lower the crib mattress to the lowest position.

- Immediately remove and replace a cracked plastic teething rail.

- Never use thin plastic bags to cover mattresses or pillows or to store bedding.

- Do not put a pillow in the crib of an infant. Save it until the child transfers into a bed.

- Place only small soft toys in a crib; large ones can be stood upon and can lead to a fall.

- Stop using the crib once the height of the top rails is less than three-fourths of the child's height, usually when the child reaches about 35 inches.

- Place an infant on the side or back for sleep to possibly reduce the risk of a sudden infant death.

High Chairs

High chairs allow children to explore food and to feed themselves with a minimum of kitchen mess. However, adult supervision is necessary.

Your responsibility checklist includes:

- Never leave a child unattended in a high chair.

- Use a high chair with both a lap and a crotch strap. Always fasten the straps. From the first

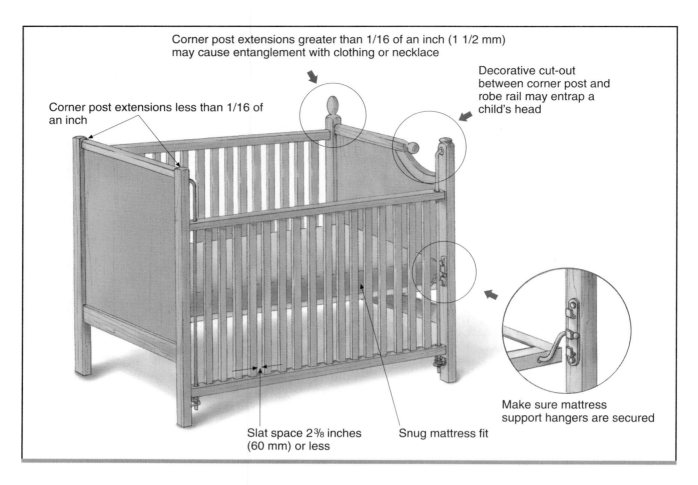

Corner post extensions greater than 1/16 of an inch (1 1/2 mm) may cause entanglement with clothing or necklace

Decorative cut-out between corner post and robe rail may entrap a child's head

Corner post extensions less than 1/16 of an inch

Make sure mattress support hangers are secured

Slat space 2⅜ inches (60 mm) or less

Snug mattress fit

time the high chair is introduced, the child must understand that being safely secured is part of the eating process.

- If your high chair is old or straps are missing, purchase a safety harness and leave it attached to the chair.

- If the seat feels slippery, attach rough-surfaced adhesive strips.

- If the high chair has a detachable tray, teach the child to raise hands over the head while you attach or detach the tray to prevent pinched fingers.

- Do not allow a child to climb into a high chair unassisted nor to stand on the seat.

- Position the high chair away from the table, countertop, stove, or electric or phone cords and out of the busy area of the kitchen.

- When using a portable high chair that attaches to a table, use one that locks on the table with a vise-like grip. Pull on the chair to be certain that it is firmly attached before seating a child. As a child grows, be aware of the seat's weight limit. Always fasten the crotch/lap belt. Avoid placing it on the side of a table near the flow of

traffic. Do not attach it to a table with a center pedestal base.

Playpens

Playpens can provide a safe play environment when there are tasks or other children that require your full attention.

Your responsibility checklist includes:

- Check that the weave of the mesh-netting walls is tiny enough so that small items cannot be pushed into the playpen by other children.

- Do not place large toys in a playpen. Children can stand on these and fall out over the siderails.

- Do not hang toys with cords across the playpen because of the risk of strangulation.

- Remove the playpen once the child is able to climb over the side.

- Never leave the sides of a mesh playpen in the down position. Infants can suffocate by becoming trapped between the mesh sides and the thin plastic mattress.

- Measure the slats on an older wooden playpen to be sure that they are no more than 2⅜ inches apart. If the space between slats is larger, there is a risk that the child will become trapped between them.

Walkers and Saucers

Walkers enable older infants to walk around before they have mastered this task on their own. In fact, it is surprising how fast an infant can propel a walker. Unfortunately, many injuries to infants have occurred as a result of this speed along with the access to unsafe areas and items that a walker provides. In addition, they are easily tipped over on any surface other than a smooth one.

Walkers can be used safely if you follow the detailed instructions concerning their safe use that accompany the packaging. Put a child in a walker only at a time when you can give your full attention to the activity.

Manufacturers also offer walker-like, stationary exercisers called saucers that spin, bounce, and rock and look very much like a walker but eliminate the ability to move around. While saucers are safer than walkers, some experts caution that both should be used for only short periods of time. This is because both saucers and walkers place children in an upright position before their muscles are ready, setting up incorrect postural alignment and allowing them to hyperextend their backs.

Your responsibility checklist includes:

- Select a walker with a wide wheelbase. This increases stability and reduces the chance of tipping.
- To prevent pinched fingers, select a walker with protective covers over the scissor component and coil springs.
- Properly prepare a safe area for the infant to explore in the walker by securing stairways, closing the bathroom and other doors, and removing objects from low tables and bookshelves.
- Keep the walker on a smooth, flat surface. Edges of rugs on wooden floors and raised door thresholds are examples of uneven surfaces that increase the chance of tipping.
- Do not use a walker on a deck, sidewalk or driveway, ramp, grass, or gravel.
- Constantly supervise an infant in a walker.
- Retrieve toys that fall to the floor because, in some models, there is an increased risk of

tipping when an infant leans too far over to one side trying to pick up a dropped toy.

Choking Prevention and Food

Choking is one of the leading causes of death to children and is most often experienced by children under the age of 3. Food is the most common cause of choking. Read about emergency care for choking, or airway obstruction, in Chapter 3.

Follow these safety rules regarding food to prevent choking:

- Teach children that it is important not to speak with food in the mouth. A laugh or sudden gasp can direct food into the airway.
- Make certain that children always sit while eating.
- Cut up or break food into small manageable pieces.
- Avoid giving the following foods to children under the age of 1 and give them with close supervision to children between the ages of 1 and 3:

  Apple peels
  Baby food meat sticks
  Bony fish
  Chewing gum
  Corn kernels
  Croissant rolls

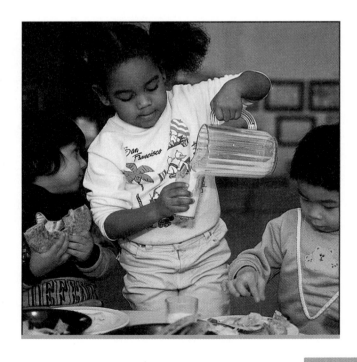

Grapes (unless cut in half)

Hard candy

Hotdogs

Ice

Marshmallows

Nuts

Oranges

Peanut butter (unless thinned with juice or milk)

Popcorn

Raisins

Raw carrot sticks

Raw celery sticks

Toy Safety

Government regulations on newly manufactured toys reduce potential hazards and help to maintain high standards for American-made toys. These regulations, together with good faith compliance and conscientious testing by the industry, make toys for today's children much safer than those of the generation before them. However, not all toy-related injuries can be prevented by government regulations and the toy industry.

Toy manufacturers label toys with children's age recommendations and, although they are sound recommendations, they are only *their* guide. You know the children well. Consider their developmental stages, their style of play, and interests. Do they play vigorously? Do they mouth toys?

The following are guidelines for preventing toy injuries:

- Read labels. Look for manufacturers' age recommendations. Only allow young children to play with toys or toy parts that are too large to become lodged in the back of the throat.

- Check each toy carefully, making sure that no small part can be pulled off. Check for sharp points or edges, exposed wires, and torn seams.

- Choose toys that hold up well to repetitive use.

- Discard plastic packaging immediately.

- Never repair toys for a young child who tends to throw toys or mouth them. Discard broken toys immediately.

- Sand wooden toys if they have any rough edges.

- Be cautious in purchasing brightly painted toys from foreign markets because many are painted with lead-containing paint.

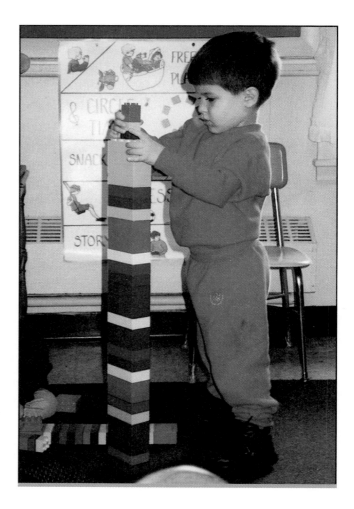

- Keep uninflated balloons and small balloon pieces out of the reach of children.

- Teach children to keep loud toys away from their ears and those of others.

- Purchase only nontoxic crayons, paints, and other art supplies.

- Teach children to put toys away. Toys left on the floor become a safety hazard.

- Store toys in plastic storage containers or in toy boxes with plastic lids and air holes or spring-loaded hinges that support the lid in any position. Heavy, free-falling lids are responsible for many injuries.

- In households with children of different ages, store toys with small parts for older children separately from toys for younger children.

- Do not allow a child to dress up in a cape or scarf that touches the floor. It might injure the child's neck if someone steps on it from behind.

- Teach older children that their electric toys, chemistry sets, and hobby items are unsafe for young children and should never be left where they can reach them.

- Use adult toys, such as lawn darts, dart guns, and bows and arrows, only when children are not present.
- Make sure that batteries in toys are inaccessible to the child.

For infants:

- Use only rattles and squeeze toys that are too large to become lodged in the back of the infant's throat.
- Do not hang toys with long cords or strings in or across a crib or playpen due to the risk of strangulation. Remove long ribbons or strings from stuffed animals. Also see *Cribs*.
- Do not hang pacifiers on cords or ribbons around a child's neck. Use pacifiers with ventilation holes and a guard shield that is too large to fit inside the mouth.
- Use with caution the doorway-mounted jumpers with canvas or fabric seats that allow an infant to bounce in place. Never leave the child unattended and use for only short periods of time.

Playground and Outdoor Safety

The U.S. Consumer Product Safety Commission reports that approximately 400,000 children are injured each year on the nation's playgrounds and that 25% of these injuries are treated in hospitals. An estimated 20 children die every year as a result of a playground injury.

Safety guidelines for playgrounds include the following:

- Be certain that there is sand, pea gravel, mulch, or a mat under all climbing equipment and swings.
- Use playgrounds where the swing area is separate from the other playground equipment to reduce the chance of a child running too close and being struck by a swing.
- Swing seats should be sling-style and made from canvas or hard rubber. Avoid seats made of metal or wood to minimize the severity of an injury to a child who is struck by an empty swing seat. Sling-style seats also discourage children from trying to swing standing up.
- Use the bucket-style swing for a toddler whenever possible.

- Proper slide safety includes: keeping one arm's length between each other on the stairs, climbing up the steps rather than up the slide, and one child at a time sliding feet first and immediately moving away from the bottom of the slide.

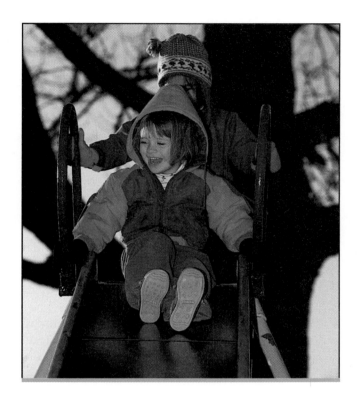

- During hot weather, check a metal slide with your hand before you allow a child to slide down. If in direct sun, a metal slide can be too hot to use safely during part of the day.
- Slides and climbing structures should be no higher than 6 feet for children under age 8 years, and a maximum of 8 feet is recommended for all children.
- Allow children on a seesaw only if the structure is affixed in sand, pea gravel, or pine bark mulch and then only with supervision. Teach them about the importance of keeping legs and heads out from under the seat.
- Do not lift a child to reach a climbing structure. If it is too high for the child to reach, it is too big and possibly too advanced for the child's ability.
- Sand box areas should be raked regularly for debris and to turn over and dry out the sand. Always cover a back yard sand box to keep cats and wild animals out of it.
- Fence in your outdoor home play area.

- Place plastic caps over protruding sharp ends and screws if you have a metal swing set.

- Inspect wooden climbing structures routinely, and sand rough areas to prevent splinters.

- Do not allow children to play behind parked cars in the driveway.

Bicycle Safety

Bicycle riding is good exercise and is enjoyed by people of all ages. However, bicycles are associated with a high number of accidents and injuries. The U.S. Consumer Product Safety Commission has issued safety regulations for bicycle manufacturers to eliminate or reduce risks of injury associated with design, construction, and performance. Yet this solves only part of the problem. Adults, whether supervising child riders or cycling with child passengers, must always keep safety in mind. For safety guidelines for older children on bicycles, see Chapter 18, *As Children Grow*.

Safety guidelines for younger children include:

- Have a tricycle available that fits the child today, not one to grow into later. A tricycle that is too large can be hard to control, and one that is too small can be unstable under a vigorous rider.

- Consider using the style of tricycle with the seat low to the ground and at the same level as the pedals. This style is more stable than the models that have a high seat and low pedals.

- Allow only one child at a time to use a tricycle.

- Ride on flat surfaces only and not on streets where motorists might have difficulty seeing the child and tricycle.

- Check tricycles for wear, sharp edges, and loose or missing parts. Store tricycles in a garage or under cover overnight to prevent rust, which ages and weakens the metal.

Safety guidelines for a child passenger on an adult bike include:

- Passenger bicycle seats are recommended for use beginning at the age of 1 year. When purchasing a bicycle seat, choose a model whose seat back extends high enough to protect the child's head; the seat should also come with protective plastic that covers the bicycle spokes to prevent feet from getting caught in them. Do not buy a used bicycle seat if any of the parts are missing.

- Make certain that the child always wears a properly fitting helmet.

- Readjust the seat belt so that the closure is on the outside back of the seat instead of across the lap. Only you can then unbuckle it.

- Remember that the additional weight of the child requires more energy from the adult pedaling and makes the bicycle less stable. Braking time is increased and downhill cruising speeds can increase without your noticing.

- Pick safe routes. Do not bike in inclement weather, when visibility is reduced, wet tires skid, and wet hand brakes do not work effectively.

Car Safety

Car accidents are, by far, the leading cause of injury and death in children from ages 1 to 14. Most children injured or killed in motor vehicle accidents are not restrained in car seats or seat belts. All 50 states, the District of Columbia, and Puerto Rico have child passenger safety laws making it illegal and punishable by a fine to transport a child in a vehicle without a car seat restraint or properly adjusted seat belt. Restrained children are less likely to distract the driver and more likely to nap or look at books and toys. A child who uses a safety restraint from infancy is not aware of any other way to travel and, as the child grows, is more likely to accept car restraints as a way of life.

Did You Know?

In a 30-mph car accident, an unrestrained child hits the dashboard or windshield with the same force as falling from a third-floor window.

Child safety seats come in a variety of sizes and styles. Choose one that is easy to use and one that fits properly in the car; use it exactly as the manufacturer instructs every time you get into the car. A car seat used part-time is risky. A car seat used improperly is as dangerous as no restraint at all. There are also specially-made car seats and car beds available for medically fragile children and premature infants.

Your responsibility checklist includes the following:

- Teach children beginning in infancy that buckling up is the first step in starting the car. As an adult, you set an example for children by your attitude towards seat belts and your consistency in using them.

- Use a car seat that meets or exceeds government safety standards. Secure infants weighing up to 20 pounds in an infant safety seat facing backwards. Secure toddlers or children weighing between 20 and 40 pounds in a safety seat facing forward. Secure children weighing between 40 pounds and 70 pounds in a car booster seat. Children who are this size have outgrown safety seats but are not big or tall enough for the adult-sized restraint. A booster seat incorporates the adult lap belt and shoul-

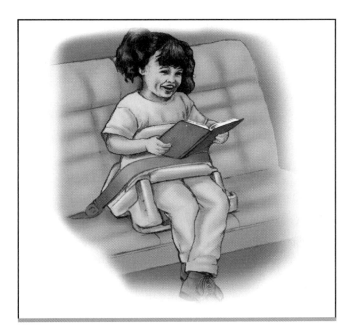

Booster seat

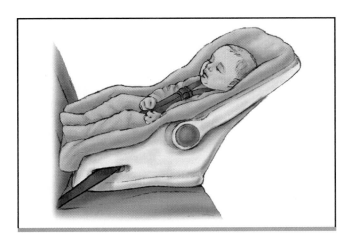

Infant car seat (infant faces seat)

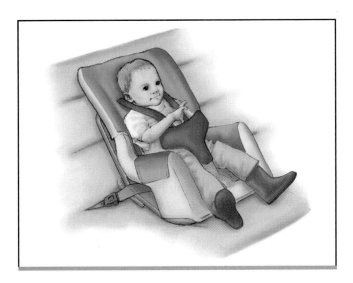

Toddler car seat (toddler faces front of car)

der restraint. Some models have a padded shield in front of the child. The child should use the booster seat until large enough for the adult lap belt to rest across the pelvis, not the abdomen. If the belt rests across the child's abdomen, it could result in a serious internal injury in a collision. Some cars have a child restraint system built into the center back seat.

- Place a child's car seat in the center of the back seat as often as possible because it is the safest location for a child passenger.

- Never substitute a household booster seat for the car booster seat nor an infant play seat for an infant car seat.

- There must be one seat belt for every child. Do not allow children to share seat belts because the impact of a collision can crush one child against the other.

- Do not permit a child to ride on an adult's lap. An unrestrained child will be thrown from the adult's arms by the force of a crash. A child restrained on an adult's lap in the same belt as the adult will be crushed between the belt and the adult.

- Never allow a child to stand up while you are driving. A slight swerve or sudden stop could throw a child against the door or the dashboard.

- Do not allow a child to sit on a driver's lap to pretend to drive or to play with the car controls.

- Always lock doors securely.

- Teach children to always exit the car on the curb side and to cross in front of the car, not behind it.

- Never leave a child alone in a car.

- Remove the cigarette lighter.

- If the car has been in the sun in hot weather, touch the metal clasps of the child's car seat to check the temperature. Make sure that the child's skin does not touch hot metal.

- Keep a survival kit in the vehicle's trunk. It should include a blanket, flares, change for telephone calls, a flashlight, and batteries.

Pedestrian Safety

Short walks near home or to and from a playground provide opportunities to teach safe behavior on streets and sidewalks. Children should walk holding your hand or holding onto loops on a travel rope when walking in a group of children. A travel rope is made by tying plastic bracelets a few feet apart along a length of rope. Children are taught to always hold onto the bracelet while walking.

Include this safety teaching when walking outdoors with your children:

- Teach children to stop just before the curb or edge of the road and to wait for an adult. Never step into the street until told that it is safe to go.

- Talk about traffic, pedestrian lights, signs, and symbols so that the children learn to recognize them.

- Teach children that vehicles can injure them.

- Teach how to look for vehicles when crossing an intersection.

- Teach children that people stay on the sidewalks, while vehicles stay on the street.

Child Passengers and Air Bags

It has been known for some time that the safest place for infants and for children under age 12 in a motor vehicle is in the rear seat, properly restrained. A new concern about the danger to children who come in contact with a deploying air bag has led the National Highway Safety Transportation Administration to recommend that infants or children under age 12 never ride in the front passenger seat if the car is equipped with a passenger-side air bag.

Air bags were designed to strike the chest of an average-size male. Injury data suggest that children are particularly vulnerable to severe brain and spinal injuries from air bags deploying at the speed of approximately 200 mph and striking them in the face. A number of infants and children have been killed by inflating air bags.

Many parents, however, are concerned about the safety of placing their infant in a rear-facing car seat in the back seat. The American Academy of Pediatrics stresses that a healthy infant buckled properly in a rear-facing car seat is safe and that the risk of injury from an air bag is much greater than the risk that the infant will develop a serious health problem requiring the driver's immediate attention. Parents are urged to place infants in either front-facing or rear-facing models in the back seat. A smaller-than-average 12-year-old should continue to ride in the back seat.

- Teach children to stay away from parked vehicles on the street and in driveways.

- Teach children to cross in front of a car or bus, not behind it, when exiting from the vehicle.

- Remind older children, who may cross streets regularly, not to be distracted by conversation with friends when crossing intersections.

Water Safety

Children are attracted to water whether in a swimming pool, wading pool, bath tub, or a bucket. They are attracted to the light reflecting off a pool, they like the sound of the water running into the bathtub, and they want to get their hands in a bucket of water to splash. Unfortunately, drowning is second only to motor vehicle accidents in the number of accidental deaths to children under the age of 5 years.

A drowning can occur in only a few inches of water. Household bathtubs are a common location for infant drowning. Every year several thousand children are treated in hospital emergency rooms or are admitted for long-term care because of near-drowning injuries. This ever-present concern for safety in and around the water should keep the supervising adult constantly alert to the children's activity. Reduce the risk of injury in your child care

Did You Know?

Approximately 300 children drown each year in neighborhood pools.

Source: Center for Environmental Health and Injury Control, Centers for Disease Control

center wading pool or in your home pool by following these guidelines:

- If you own a pool, learn CPR.
- Keep your eyes on the children when around water. Never leave them unsupervised in a bathtub or any size pool, no matter how shallow the water or how short the time.

- Make certain that an adult is always present when a wading pool or bathtub is being filled.
- Empty wading pools, bathtubs, and water buckets immediately after each use.
- Keep the toilet lid down.
- Arrange for a child to learn to swim at a young age. Teach the child respect for water.
- Keep rescue flotation devices near an in-ground pool.
- Use caution in allowing nonswimmers to use a flotation device, including kickboards, in deep water. Even a momentary loss of grip on the object can cause panic and lead to drowning.
- Remove a ladder from an above-ground pool when not in use.
- Make certain that gates around a pool are securely locked when not in use. If neighbors have pools, make certain that they know that you care for children and discuss your safety issues with them.
- When you become aware that a child is missing, check the pools in the neighborhood first.
- Never leave a child alone near a frozen body of water.

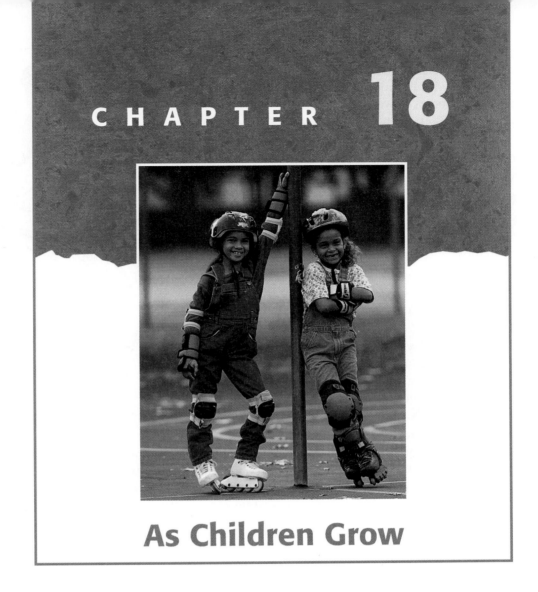

CHAPTER 18

As Children Grow

When children are very young, childproofing is absolutely necessary. This means that parents or other trusted adults must make the world safe for the curious and exploring child who is too young to understand dangers or to make safe choices on his or her own. As children grow, they leave this carefully controlled environment and must be taught to safely negotiate all of the experiences at school, on the playground, at home, or in someone else's home when an adult might not be present.

As children grow, you must warn them of hazards that they might encounter. You will, undoubtedly, establish rules for them to follow on the basis of where you live and what their activities are. Share with them the following safety rules for older children as they begin to do more for themselves at home and are exposed to more choices away from home.

Sports and at Play

- Learn how to swim. If swimming is not a favorite activity, at least know how to tread water and float on your back for your own safety. Learn the drownproofing techniques that keep a person afloat while conserving energy.

- Never swim alone. Never swim in dangerous water, such as in a quarry or near a reservoir dam, even with friends. Swim in lifeguard-protected bodies of water.

- Find out how deep the water is before diving. Never dive into shallow water, because you can break your neck if you hit the bottom forcefully.

- Wear a life jacket when boating or water skiing.

- Never walk or ice skate alone on a frozen body of water.

- Never run into the street chasing a ball, a pet, or friends.

- Do not play in unsafe areas, such as in the street, behind cars in a driveway, at a construction area, on railroad tracks, or in an abandoned building.

- Only play on playground equipment that has sand or mulch under the equipment. Never play on a playground with a concrete or asphalt surface. Serious head injuries and broken bones occur more easily here.

- If you use a seesaw, do not stand or walk on the seat board. Do not allow your feet to go under the seesaw as it hits the ground.

- When roller blading or skateboarding, wear your bike helmet. Also wear protective padding and wrist braces, and skate on flat smooth surfaces only.

Bicycle Riding

- Ride a bicycle that fits you today, not one that you will grow into later. A bicycle that is too large makes steering and braking especially difficult.

- Wear clothing designed for biking. Always wear a bike helmet to reduce the risk of serious head and brain injury in the event of a fall or a collision. Keep shoe laces tied and wear leg bands on loose-fitting pant legs to reduce the risk of clothing entanglement in the chain or sprocket.

- Do not ride your bike in bare feet.

- Ride your bicycle on the right side of the road and obey traffic signs.

- Be alert for car doors that can open unexpectedly in your path.

- Do not hang onto a moving vehicle when on a bicycle, skateboard, roller blades, or skates.

- Do not give a ride to a friend on the handlebars or on the fender of your bicycle.

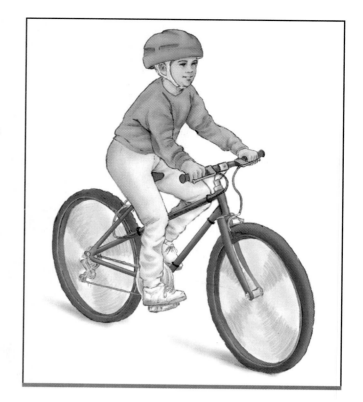

- Ride on bike paths whenever possible. If you must use roads, make sure to obey the basic bicycle rules: Bikers travel in a single file, on the right-hand side of the road, in the same direction as motor vehicle traffic. They use correct hand signals and obey all traffic lights and signs for motorists. Bikers also watch for opening car doors and for cars pulling out of driveways and parking spaces.

- Bikes should be used only in daylight and in dry weather. In bad weather, visibility is reduced, wet tires skid, and wet handbrakes do not work effectively. Reflectors should be attached in the correct locations. Riding after sunset is dangerous, even in dry weather with lights and reflectors.

- Do not clown around or perform stunts while riding your bike.

Electricity and Fire

- Never go near a downed or broken power line. The line might still be live and could kill anyone who gets too close to it. Never play near or climb on the fencing around an electricity substation. Never climb an electric utility pole.

- Never touch an electrical appliance, even if turned off, if your hands or feet are wet because

Bicycle Helmets Make Sense

- Bicycle injuries are the most common cause of sports or recreational injury in the United States.*

- More than 900 children are killed each year as the result of bicycle accidents, and another 500,000 are seen in emergency rooms. One study showed that three of every four children who are hospitalized for a bicycle injury do not wear helmets even after recovery.**

- The use of approved bicycle helmets reduces the risk of severe head injuries by 85%.***

- 75% of all fatalities in bicycle-related accidents are the result of brain injury.*

- In a bicycle accident you have a 50/50 chance of hitting your head.*

- A fall from a bicycle that is moving at 20 mph will likely result in death if the rider's head hits the pavement, rocks, or another solid object.*

Sources: *Injury Prevention Resource and Research Center, Dartmouth Medical School.
**National Head Injury Foundation. Taken from an article in Washington Post Health Section, October 16, 1990.
***National Safety Council.

of the risk of electrocution. This includes not using a hair blow dryer or other electrical appliance while in the bathtub or shower. You can be electrocuted if a plugged-in appliance touches the water.

- Never throw water on a plugged-in electrical appliance that is on fire, because of the risk of electrocution.

- Never stick anything other than an electrical plug into a wall outlet.

- Always hold on to the rubber finger grip at the base of a plug when inserting it into or unplugging it from an electrical outlet. Never touch the metal prongs. Never pull on the cord to unplug it.

- Never fly a kite or hold onto a metalized mylar balloon near an electric power line. Mylar balloons are safest when enjoyed indoors.

- Do not play with matches, lighters, or fireworks. Knowing that many children your age suffer terrible burns and other injuries from such activities should make the fun not worth the risk.

- If bread gets stuck in the toaster, do not try to get it out with a metal fork while the toaster is plugged in. Unplug the toaster before retrieving the toast.

- If food catches on fire in the microwave, turn off the microwave and leave the door closed; the fire will go out.

- Always tie back long hair when cooking over an open fire.

Personal Safety

- Do not walk toward a stranger to accept food, other gifts, or if asked for help or directions. Adults who need assistance should find another adult.

- When crossing a street, do not be distracted by conversation or by fooling around with friends. Pay attention to the traffic.

- If walking at dusk or later, always wear white because it shows up well for drivers passing by you. If there is no sidewalk, walk on the left side of the road, facing the traffic, and stay as far back from the edge of the road as you can.

- At the first rumble of thunder, get out of water. Preferably, find protection inside a building if nearby, or inside a hard-top car. Avoid being the tallest thing in the area.

- If you become completely lost in the woods, find one spot that offers some shelter and wait to be rescued. Running from place to place increases the chance of being missed by adults searching for you.

- Never put your tongue against anything metal when outside during freezing weather, because it will stick and you will be injured if you try to pull it free. The same is true for inside the freezer.

- Never put your fingers into the garbage disposal, even if it is not running.

- Never get into or put anyone inside a car trunk or old refrigerator, because not enough air can get inside and the person might suffocate.

- Never inhale the fumes of a chemical because someone told you how good it feels to "get high." It is extremely dangerous to your brain, liver, and nervous system.

- Ride only on the inside of a vehicle. Do not ride on the bumpers, hood, trunk, or other exterior surfaces.

- Always buckle your car seat belt, even if others in the car do not.

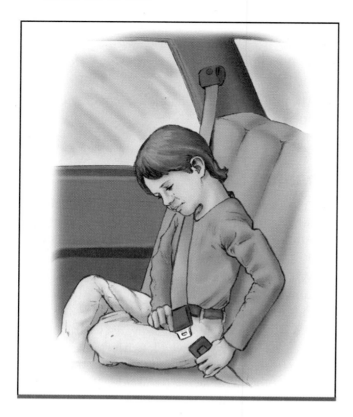

- Never, never get in a car if the driver has been drinking alcohol or using drugs.

Firearms Safety

It is estimated that almost half of American homes with children have one or more handguns. Homicides are a leading cause of injury-related death in children under the age of 18, followed by suicide. The National Center for Health Statistics reports that every day in America, 16 children under the age of 20 are killed in gun homicides, suicides, and unintentional shootings and that many more suffer wounds. Approximately 66% of all homicides and more than half of all suicides among children involve handguns. In addition, approximately 16% of all unintentional firearm deaths occur in children under the age of 18 who were "just fooling around when it went off."

The increased availability and use of handguns can only ensure that the number of children injured and killed by them will continue to rise. Children alone at home after school with access to firearms

present an unknown potential for serious injury and death.

Children are curious by nature and the lure of the forbidden when a firearm is accessible creates the potential for a disaster. Few children under the age of 8 can reliably tell the difference between a real gun and a toy gun. The noticeable difference in weight between a real gun and a toy gun does not register as an important indicator of danger in the mind of a child. Children should play with only brightly-colored toy guns, so that they can clearly understand the difference between what is play and what can kill. Parents might consider disposing of toy guns that look identical to real ones.

Even if parents do not own a firearm, it is worthwhile finding out if firearms are present in the homes of their relatives and their children's friends. This suggestion is based on a study of unintentional handgun shootings of children under age 16 that found that nearly 40% of these shootings occurred in the homes of relatives and friends. Most of these tragedies occurred when children were not supervised. No firearm should ever be present in a child care center or in a house or apartment where home-based child care is provided.

Pump air guns, air rifles, air pistols, and BB guns can also cause injuries and deaths. Projectiles from these weapons can reach speeds comparable to some handguns and can penetrate skin and bone.

The best way to remove the risk of gun violence to children is to remove firearms from the home entirely. In a home in which there is a firearm, there is always some risk of injury to a child. If you must own a firearm, consider the following guidelines for the safe storage and care of it.

- Store the firearm unloaded and locked in a cabinet. For a revolver, open the cylinder and place a pad lock around the top strap to prevent it from closing. For a pistol, use a trigger lock on the trigger.

- Store ammunition separately from the firearm in a locked location.

- Do not let anyone under the age of 18 know where the keys are kept or the firearm is stored.

- Never leave a firearm unattended.

- If the firearm is ever in their presence, demonstrate for children that it should always be handled as if loaded and never pointed at anyone.

Common Childhood Illnesses

Listed alphabetically, the following chart of symptoms or health complaints that a child might describe provides information about several illnesses and health conditions commonly experienced by children. Each symptom provides recommendations helpful to child care providers and to parents, and many topics suggest common, but not all diagnoses for the symptom.

Anal Itching

Possible Diagnosis: Pinworms

What You Should Know
- An intestinal parasitic worm infection
- Acquired by ingesting microscopic pinworm eggs after outdoor play in dirt or sand
- Common among young children who often have their hands in their mouths, and are poor hand washers
- Can cause intense rectal/anal itching
- Highly contagious in a family or child care setting
- Spreads to others when child scratches anal area, getting eggs under fingernails, and then touches another's food or other items that might be mouthed. Also spreads from eggs on pajamas, linens, underpants, etc.
- Diagnosed with special pinworm kit used by parent to collect parasite specimen from anal skin

What You Can Do As a Caregiver
- Discourage scratching anal area
- Encourage child to wash hands after outdoor play
- Notify parent

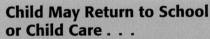

Child May Return to School or Child Care . . .
after child has been treated initially and after itching subsides.

What You Can Do As a Parent
- Follow Caregiver recommendations
- Trim fingernails short
- Wash child's bed linen, clothing, and towels in hot water and dry on high heat setting; do not shake items because this will scatter the eggs

Constipation

What You Should Know
- Defined as hard stools that cause painful elimination
- Can be caused by diet low in fiber and inadequate fluid intake
- Sometimes caused by postponing or resisting urge to eliminate

Child May Return to School or Child Care . . .
child need not be excluded from child care or school.

What You Can Do As a Caregiver
- Encourage child to drink clear fluids
- Encourage child to eat foods that contain fiber and have a tendency to soften the stool, such as whole grains, peaches, prunes, grapes, raisins, plums, melons, carrots, celery, and lettuce
- Reduce intake of foods that bind, such as milk, hard cheese, cottage cheese, bananas, apples, applesauce, and white-flour baked goods
- Encourage a regular toileting

What You Can Do As a Parent
- Follow Caregiver recommendations
- Call child's health care provider if problem persists for several weeks

Coughing

What You Should Know
- A symptom of an irritation within the respiratory tract
- Often accompanies a viral infection, such as a cold
- Also see *Croup,* Chapter 12

What You Can Do As a Caregiver
- Encourage child to cover mouth, and wash hands thoroughly and often
- See *Colds,* Chapter 16, and *Preventing Infection in a Child Care Setting,* Chapter 15

What You Can Do As a Parent
- Follow Caregiver recommendations
- Notify child's health care provider if child develops a fever, or if cough persists for longer than 1 week

Child May Return to School or Child Care . . .
child need not be excluded from child care or school unless cough is accompanied by fever.

Possible Diagnosis: Pertussis (Whooping cough)

What You Should Know
- Commonly known as "whooping cough" because of the whooping noise a child makes when coughing
- Highly contagious bacterial infection
- Spreads to others through coughing and sneezing
- Incubation period averages 7 to 10 days
- Illness generally mild in older children, but can be life-threatening to infants because of breathing difficulties, pneumonia, and brain swelling
- First stage of infection lasts approximately 1 week and mimics the usual cold symptoms of runny nose, sneezing, and coughing, which can delay diagnosis
- Second stage lasts approximately 4 to 6 weeks, with uncontrollable coughing spells, often accompanied by whooping noise when child inhales. Cough can be so violent that it causes vomiting. Child may cough up thick mucus.
- Diagnosed by nasal culture within first 2 weeks of coughing and with a blood test if cough has lasted longer than 2 weeks
- Treated with antibiotics for 14 days
- Vaccine is given to infants as part of DPT (diptheria, pertussis, tetanus) immunization to protect young children, but immunity diminishes as years pass
- A pertussis infection gives lifelong immunity
- Centers for Disease Control requires all health care providers and state medical labs to report positive results for pertussis on cultures to the Department of Public Health

What You Can Do As a Caregiver
- Encourage parent of child with prolonged cough to take child to health care provider
- Alert other parents if a child is diagnosed with pertussis. Encourage them to contact their health care providers. Maintain confidentiality.
- For more information, contact your local Department of Public Health

Child May Return to School or Child care . . .
after the first 5 days of 14-day antibiotic treatment course.

What You Can Do As a Parent
- Have child seen by health care provider for prolonged cough

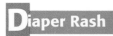

Possible Diagnosis: **Simple diaper rash**

What You Should Know
- Commonly occurs when bacteria in bowel react with urine to form ammonia, which irritates and burns skin
- Prolonged exposure to soiled diaper and friction against skin worsens rash
- Can be painful

What You Can Do As a Caregiver
- Change diapers often; wear disposable gloves
- Wash diaper area with soap and warm water; allow complete drying
- Place child in cool baths with ½ cup vinegar for 15 to 20 minutes, several times per day. Vinegar reduces bacterial growth and helps to neutralize ammonia.
- Protect diaper area with over-the-counter ointments, such as zinc oxide or petroleum jelly, which act as moisture barriers
- Wash hands thoroughly after removing gloves
- Do not use baby powder on diaper area because child might inhale talc
- Cloth diapers should be washed commercially, or presoaked in mild vinegar water before washing, to remove ammonia

Child May Return to School or Child Care . . . child need not be excluded from child care or school.

What You Can Do As a Parent
- Follow Caregiver recommendations

Possible Diagnosis: **Candida infection**

What You Should Know
- Caused by a yeast infection within the intestines
- Appears as a fiery red rash
- Can be spread from child to child by an adult who does not wash hands thoroughly
- Treated with prescription medication
- Infection can also be present in mouth
- Also see *Thrush* under *Mouth/Lip Eruptions* (caused by same organism)

What You Can Do As a Caregiver
- Change diapers often; wear disposable gloves
- Wash diaper area with soap and warm water; allow complete drying
- Do not use baby powder on diaper area because child might inhale talc
- Wash hands thoroughly after removing gloves

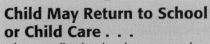

Child May Return to School or Child Care . . . when medication has been started.

What You Can Do As a Parent
- Follow Caregiver recommendations
- Call child's health care provider for prescription ointment and discuss treatment with oral medication

Diarrhea

What You Should Know
- Defined as several loose or watery stools
- Caused primarily by viruses
- Can also be caused by bacterial infections, antibiotics, and certain foods
- Most noninfectious diarrhea resolves without treatment within a few days
- If mild diarrhea does not resolve within a few days, child should be seen by health care provider for stool culture to determine if diarrhea is infectious

What You Can Do As a Caregiver
- See *Diarrhea*, Chapter 16, and *Preventing Infection in a Child Care Setting*, Chapter 15

What You Can Do as a Parent
- Follow Caregiver recommendations

Possible Diagnosis: Infectious diarrhea

What You Should Know
- An intestinal infection caused by bacteria such as *Salmonella* and *Shigella* species, a parasite such as *Giardia*, or a virus
- Varies from mild to severe
- Signs and symptoms:
    - Diarrhea containing blood or mucus
    - Stomach or abdominal cramping and gas
    - Foul-smelling stools
    - Fever
    - Weight loss
- Acquired by ingestion of contaminated water or food
- Highly contagious
- Diagnosed by stool culture(s)
- Treated with prescription medication
- Infection should be reported to your local Department of Public Health by your child's health care provider

What You Can Do As a Caregiver
- Wear disposable gloves for diapering or helping with toileting to reduce chances of infection spreading. Wash hands thoroughly after removing gloves.
- Encourage child to drink an extra amount of clear fluids
- Do not allow child to share drinking glass or eating utensils with others
- Discuss treatment of all family members with health care provider
- See *Diarrhea*, Chapter 16, and *Preventing Infection in a Child Care Setting*, Chapter 15

What You Can Do As a Parent
- Follow Caregiver recommendations
- Contact child's health care provider

Possible Diagnosis: Hepatitis A

What You Should Know
- An infection of the liver caused by a virus found in the intestines, and spread through the stool; not necessarily diarrhea
- Virus spreads from person to person when hands contaminated with microscopic particles of stool touch food or eating utensils
- Mild flu-like symptoms develop 2 to 8 weeks after exposure
- Contagious for 2 weeks before symptoms develop
- Illness more serious in adults than in children
- Illness should be reported to your local Department of Public Health by your health care provider
- No specific treatment

What You Can Do As a Caregiver
- See *Infectious diarrhea*
- Contact your health care provider if you are exposed to the Hepatitis A virus

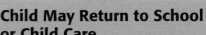

Child May Return to School or Child Care . . .
child need not be excluded from child care or school if diarrhea can be contained in diaper or by normal toileting practices.

Child May Return to School or Child Care . . .
if *Salmonella*: After treatment with antibiotics, and after 3 negative results on stool cultures. If *Shigella*: After treatment with antibiotics, after severe diarrhea is under control, and child is able to contain diarrhea with normal toileting practices. If *Giardia*: After treatment with prescription medication, after severe diarrhea is under control, and child is able to contain diarrhea with normal toileting practices. In all cases: Check with your health care consultant about your center's policy concerning a child's return after treatment for infectious diarrhea.

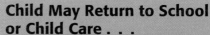

Child May Return to School or Child Care . . .
child should remain at home while ill, and may return when symptoms are no longer present, and when temperature is normal for 24 hours. Check with your health care consultant concerning a child's return following Hepatitis A infection.

What You Can Do As a Parent
- Follow Caregiver recommendations
- Contact child's health care provider if exposed to the Hepatitis A virus

Ear Pain

Possible Diagnosis: **Otitis media (Middle ear infection)**

What You Should Know
- Can be painful
- Often follows a cold that causes mucous blockage of the tube that connects throat and middle ear (eustachian tube), preventing drainage and allowing bacteria to cause infection
- Signs and symptoms:
  - Repeated pulling of ear(s)
  - Cries of pain and general irritability
  - Fever
  - Fluid draining from ear(s)
- Treated with antibiotics
- Not contagious
- Some children have ear tubes inserted through the ear drum to allow fluid and pus to drain out through ear canal. Special precautions must be taken to avoid getting water into ears during shampooing and swimming.
- Also see *Foreign Objects,* Chapter 7

What You Can Do As a Caregiver
- Take temperature and treat as necessary with acetaminophen
- Notify parent
- Hold child in upright position to decrease pressure in ear and lessen pain
- Do not allow child to drink from bottle while lying on the back, because this can encourage fluids containing mouth bacteria to enter eustachian tube and travel to middle ear
- Never insert anything, including cotton swabs, into child's ear
- Watch for hearing loss or speech problem in child with recurring ear infections

> **Child May Return to School or Child Care . . .**
> when child feels better and temperature is normal.

What You Can Do As a Parent
- Follow Caregiver recommendations
- Call child's health care provider

Eye Irritation/Pain

Possible Diagnosis: **Conjunctivitis (Pink eye)**

What You Should Know
- Infection of the lining of the eye, often accompanying a cold
- Signs and symptoms:
  - Red, irritated, or painful eye(s)
  - Yellow or watery drainage
  - Eyelids temporarily stuck together from encrusted discharge when child awakens from sleep
- Easily spread by touching infected secretions and then touching own eye area
- Watery drainage is most likely viral conjunctivitis and resolves without treatment
- Pus or yellow drainage is most likely bacterial conjunctivitis and must be treated with an antibiotic

What You Can Do As a Caregiver
- Wear disposable gloves. Clean drainage from child's eye(s) with clean tissue or gauze pad and warm water, as needed. Wipe each eye outward from inner corner. Wear disposable gloves.
- Discourage touching eye(s).
- Wash hands thoroughly and encourage child to do the same
- Notify parent if eye has pus or yellow drainage
- See *Preventing Infection in a Child Care Setting,* Chapter 15

Child May Return to School or Child Care . . . when child is comfortable and eye discharge contains no pus, or after 24 hours of antibiotic treatment.

What You Can Do As a Parent
- Follow Caregiver recommendations
- Call child's health care provider
- Wear disposable gloves. Apply ointment if prescribed: have child look upward; apply ointment to clean, cotton-tip applicator and then to inside of lower eyelid to avoid contaminating ointment tube

Possible Diagnosis: Sty

What You Should Know
- Infection of a sweat gland on the eye lid, usually near eye lashes
- Appears as a painful red pimple

What You Can Do As a Caregiver
- Wear disposable gloves
- Apply warm wash cloth to eye for 5 to 10 minutes several times per day
- Encourage child not to touch eyes
- Wash hands thoroughly and encourage child to do the same

Child May Return to School or Child Care . . . when child feels better.

What You Can Do As a Parent
- Follow Caregiver recommendations
- Call child's health care provider if no improvement

Fever

Possible Diagnosis: Viral or bacterial infection

What You Should Know
- A child with a fever should not be in a child care setting

What You Can Do As a Caregiver
- See *Fever,* Chapter 16

Child May Return to School or Child Care . . . when temperature is normal for 24 hours.

What You Can Do As a Parent
- See *Fever,* Chapter 16

Headache

What You Should Know
- Most are minor and are caused by overexertion or stress
- Might signal beginning of illness
- Might signal problem with vision

What You Can Do As a Caregiver

- Have child rest in a quiet, darkened area
- Give acetaminophen as needed. Know your center's policy about use of acetaminophen.
- Report recurring headaches to parent

What You Can Do As a Parent

- Have child rest in a quiet, darkened area
- Give acetaminophen as needed
- Call child's health care provider for recurrent headaches

Child May Return to School or Child Care . . . when child feels better.

Itching Scalp

Possible Diagnosis: Pediculosis capitas (Head lice)

What You Should Know

- Infestation by a tiny parasitic insect on the scalp and hair
- Signs and symptoms:
  - Persistent itching on scalp
  - Tiny red bites on scalp and on hairline
- Diagnosed by finding tiny yellow/white eggs, called nits, firmly attached to shaft of hair. Adult lice are harder to find.
- Nits found all along hair shaft and all over head, but especially at crown, nape of neck, and behind ears
- Nits are most easily seen and removed when hair is partially or completely dry
- Highly contagious
- Transferred from person to person by crawling lice or when children share personal items such as hats, combs, and brushes
- Not caused by uncleanliness
- Lice cannot jump or fly
- Not carried by cats or dogs
- Requires thorough treatment of all family members who have head lice at the same time
- Lice-killing shampoos are pesticides; use cautiously
- Also see *Ringworm* under *Skin Eruptions and Rashes*

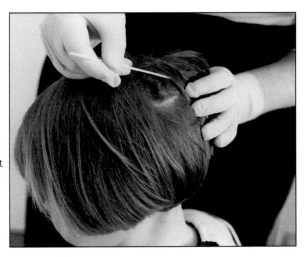

Checking for head lice

What You Can Do As a Caregiver

- Notify child's parent
- Notify all parents of a case of lice, but maintain confidentiality
- Machine wash all washable items in hot water, including bed linens, blankets, towels, clothing, jackets, and hats
- Use hot setting on dryer
- Place pillows and stuffed animals in dryer on hot setting for 30 minutes
- Place items that cannot be washed or dried in a closed plastic bag for 2 weeks
- Vacuum upholstered furniture, mattresses, rugs, car seats, and stuffed toys
- Do not use lice sprays

Child May Return to School or Child Care . . . after treatment with lice-killing shampoo and thorough nit removal. Know your center's or school's policy concerning child returning after lice infestation.

What You Can Do As a Parent

- Follow Caregiver recommendations
- Treat with lice-killing shampoo as recommended by child's health care provider. Follow package directions and wear disposable gloves when applying shampoo.
- Apply shampoo at the sink, never in the bathtub, to minimize skin exposed to pesticide
- Safest if a pregnant or nursing mother does not apply shampoo, even if wearing gloves
- Do not use lice-killing shampoo if cut or other open wound is present on scalp

- Do not use lice-killing shampoo on infants
- Treat all family members who have head lice at the same time
- Remove all nits with small metal nit comb available in most pharmacies, or with fingernails
- Check all family members' heads daily for 10 days
- May have to repeat full treatment in 1 week
- Scrub hair brushes, combs, and hair accessories, and then soak them in very hot water for 10 minutes

Mouth/Lip Eruptions

Possible Diagnosis: Cold sores (Herpes simplex virus)

What You Should Know
- A viral disease that causes recurrent infections throughout life
- Signs and symptoms:
  - Cluster of water blisters on lip
  - Can be painful
  - Blisters break, weep, and scab over in several days
- In children, the rash occurs almost exclusively on the face as a cold sore or fever blister
- Child is contagious until all blisters have scabbed
- Virus is spread by direct contact with the sore or by secretions from the sore
- Infection recurs periodically
- An adult or child who has an open herpes simplex sore on the mouth or other body area that cannot be completely covered should not be in a child care setting
- No cure available

What You Can Do As a Caregiver
- Keep area clean and dry
- Do not touch an open cold sore
- Wash hands thoroughly

What You Can Do As a Parent
- Follow Caregiver recommendations

Child May Return to School or Child Care . . .
when an open sore has completely scabbed over, or can be completely covered.

Possible Diagnosis: Hand, foot, and mouth syndrome

What You Should Know
- Mild viral infection
- Usually occurs in children between 6 months and 4 years of age
- Transmitted from person to person through saliva and stool
- Incubation period is 3 to 6 days
- Signs and symptoms:
  - Fever that is sometimes up to 104°F, lasting 3 to 4 days
  - Headache that starts about 2 days before mouth sores develop
  - Ulcer-like sores in mouth, in throat, and on tongue, making eating and drinking difficult
  - Red spots that become blisters on palms and soles
  - Rash in the groin and on buttocks that seldom blisters
- Child does not necessarily have spots or blisters in all locations
- Illness resolves on its own in about 1 week
- Typically seen in summer and fall
- Dehydration can occur in a young child who refuses to drink because of mouth sores

What You Can Do As a Caregiver
- Take child's temperature, and contact parent to pick up child
- Separate child from group

Child May Return to School or Child Care . . .
when mouth sores and blisters are healed, approximately 1 week.

What You Can Do As a Parent
- Give acetaminophen for fever over 101°F, and for pain in mouth
- Use over-the-counter products to numb mouth sores
- Rinse mouth with lukewarm water after eating
- Boil silverware or use disposable utensils to avoid transmitting disease
- Boil bottle nipples for 20 minutes
- Encourage fluids as tolerated, including popsickles; milk is often soothing
- Offer soft foods, including ice cream, sherbet, gelatin, pudding, soft breads, noodles, and rice
- Avoid citrus fruits, salty or spicy foods, carbonated beverages, crunchy cereals, and other foods requiring chewing
- Do not break blisters on hands and feet; they heal better if not broken

Possible Diagnosis: Thrush

What You Should Know
- A yeast infection in the mouth
- Appears as white patches on the mucous membranes of the mouth and on the tongue
- Easily spread from one infant to another
- Seldom occurs in infants over 6 months of age
- Must be treated with antifungal medication
- Also see *Candida infection* under *Diaper Rash*

> **Child May Return to School or Child Care . . .**
> when treatment has started.

What You Can Do As a Caregiver
- Wear disposable gloves when handling child's mouthed items to reduce the chance of infection spreading to others
- Wash hands thoroughly after removing gloves
- Carefully wash all items that might reinfect child, such as nipples, pacifier, and mouthed toys
- Do not allow babies to share mouthed toys, pacifiers, or bottles

What You Can Do As a Parent
- Follow Caregiver recommendations

Runny Nose

Possible Diagnosis: Cold (See *Colds,* Chapter 16)

Skin Eruptions and Rashes

Possible Diagnosis: Chicken pox

What You Should Know
- A common viral illness lasting approximately 1 week
- Incubation period is 10 to 21 days
- Contagious from 1 to 2 days before rash appears until all blisters have scabbed over (about 1 week)
- Rash of red bumps appears primarily on face and trunk as fluid-filled bubbles that break, weep, and scab
- Rash can also appear on arms, legs, or any mucous membrane surface, such as inside the mouth, throat, eyes, and vagina
- Other signs and symptoms:
  - Fever
  - Itching
- Is spread by nose or throat secretions containing chicken pox virus, or by touching rash
- Dry scabs are not contagious

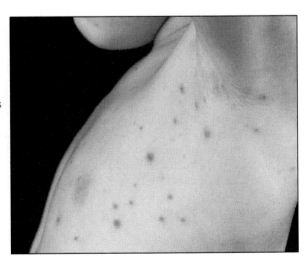

Chicken pox

- One bout provides immunity
- Vaccine available

What You Can Do As a Caregiver
- Wear disposable gloves and wash hands thoroughly after removing gloves
- Take temperature and treat for fever as necessary. Know your center's policy concerning the use of acetaminophen.
- Notify parent
- See *Fever,* Chapter 16

What You Can Do As a Parent
- Encourage child to drink clear fluids
- Bathe child in warm water with ½ cup baking soda or 1 to 2 cups colloidal oatmeal to relieve itching
- Apply calamine lotion to relieve itching; avoid eyes
- Call child's health care provider, who might recommend a medicine for itching
- Trim child's fingernails or put mittens on infant to prevent scratching, which can infect open lesions and lead to scarring
- Avoid giving aspirin
- See *Reye's Syndrome and Aspirin,* Chapter 16
- Notify child's health care provider if child is unusually uncomfortable, cannot drink, has persistent high fever, severe headache, or is disoriented
- Watch for chicken pox to develop in other family members or playmates for 3 weeks

Child May Return to School or Child Care . . . when all blisters have scabbed over, approximately 7 days

Possible Diagnosis: Fifth disease

What You Should Know
- Mild viral illness, harmless for most children
- Incubation period is 4 to 14 days
- Contagious several days before appearance of rash
- Signs and symptoms:
    - Bright red rash on cheeks, giving face a "slapped cheek" appearance
    - Lacey red rash on arms, legs, and trunk; usually gone in 10 days
- Other symptoms, which pass in a few days, include: low-grade fever, fatigue, headache, sore throat, stomachache, chills, and decreased appetite
- Rash may recur periodically over the following 3 to 4 months, usually due to sunlight, warm baths, or emotional upset; child will not be contagious
- Virus spreads through contact with throat and mouth secretions
- Can be serious for children with some chronic illnesses, such as sickle cell anemia and thalessemia, and those with suppressed immune systems, such as leukemia and AIDS patients
- May present risk to fetus
- No vaccine available
- One bout of infection is believed to provide lifelong immunity

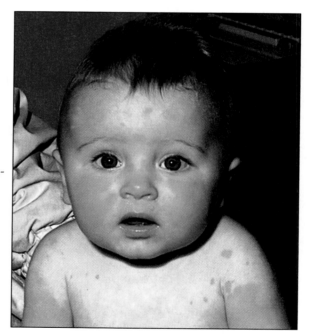

Fifth disease

What You Can Do As a Caregiver
- Wear disposable gloves and wash hands thoroughly after removing gloves
- Take temperature and treat for fever as necessary. Know your center's policy concerning the use of acetaminophen.
- Notify all parents because of possible health risks to unborn babies and to children with serious illnesses. A pregnant woman who is exposed to fifth disease should consult her health care provider.

What You Can Do As a Parent
- Give acetaminophen for fever and headache
- Contact child's health care provider

Child May Return to School or Child Care . . . child need not be excluded from child care or school if temperature is normal and child feels well.

Possible Diagnosis: Heat rash (Prickly heat)

What You Should Know
- Experienced mostly by infants and young children
- Characterized by tiny pink bumps in areas that tend to be moist
- Commonly seen in skin folds of neck and on upper chest, arms, legs, and diaper area
- Occurs during hot and humid weather
- Clears up in a few days

What You Can Do As a Caregiver
- Pay special attention to skin folds that stay wet with perspiration, urine, or drool
- Apply calamine lotion to reddest areas
- Leave areas open to air, without clothing
- Allow fan to blow gently on child when sleeping
- Do not apply skin ointments
- Use powder in sparse amounts by pouring a small amount into your hand, away from child's face, and applying to skin so powder is barely visible. Be aware that use of powder is generally not recommended for children because of risk of inhalation of talc.

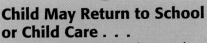

Child May Return to School or Child Care . . .
child need not be excluded from child care or school.

What You Can Do As a Parent
- Follow Caregiver recommendations
- Bathe child without soap
- Allow skin to air dry

Possible Diagnosis: Impetigo

What You Should Know
- A streptococcal or staphylococcal bacterial skin infection that can develop after an insect bite, cut, or other break in the skin
- Commonly seen on the face but can develop in any skin injury, such as insect bite or cut
- Signs and symptoms:
    - Red, oozing rash covered by fine, honey-colored scab
    - Pain and itching
- Can spread to other parts of child's body if child scratches
- Can spread to others in close contact by direct touching or touching a surface contaminated with secretions
- Requires topical antibiotic ointment
- Infection more worrisome in infants than in older children

What You Can Do As a Caregiver
- Notify parent
- Discourage scratching
- Trim fingernails
- Do not permit sharing of towels or face cloths
- Wear disposable gloves while caring for infected skin to reduce chance of infection spreading to you and others
- Wash hands thoroughly after removing gloves
- Observe rash and note any improvement or worsening

Child May Return to School or Child Care . . .
24 hours after treatment is started.

What You Can Do As a Parent
- Follow Caregiver recommendations
- Call child's health care provider for antibiotic ointment recommendation
- Remove scab by soaking before applying antibiotic ointment

Possible Diagnosis: **Ringworm**

What You Should Know

- A minor infection that is mildly contagious
- A superficial fungal infection of the skin, affecting young children primarily on the scalp and trunk
- Scalp infection causes temporary bald patches, ½ to 2 inches in diameter
- On trunk, infection causes round or oval, red, scaly patches that spread outward and heal in the center, resembling a doughnut
- Infection cannot penetrate skin but sits on the surface
- Spreads from person to person by direct contact with ringworm lesion
- Treated with antifungal topical cream that must be used for several weeks after rash disappears
- No longer contagious 48 hours after treatment

What You Can Do As a Caregiver

- Notify parent at end of day
- Wash hands thoroughly and encourage child to do the same

What You Can Do As a Parent

- Wear disposable gloves when treating with over-the-counter antifungal cream or ointment
- Continue to use cream or ointment for several weeks after rash disappears
- Wash hands thoroughly after removing gloves

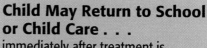

Child May Return to School or Child Care . . . immediately after treatment is started.

Possible Diagnosis: **Roseola**

What You Should Know

- A viral illness occurring in young children primarily under the age of 2 years
- Incubation period is 5 to 15 days
- Mildly contagious
- Characterized by a persistent high fever (103°F or higher) for 3 to 4 days without other symptoms
- Fever drops suddenly about day 4, and generalized red rash appears over the entire body
- Rash is gone in about 24 hours
- One bout provides immunity

What You Can Do As a Caregiver

- Take temperature and treat for fever as necessary. Know your center's policy concerning the use of acetaminophen.
- Notify parent
- Encourage clear fluids

What You Can Do As a Parent

- Call child's health care provider
- See *Fever*, in Chapter 16

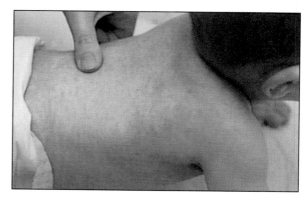

Roseola

Child May Return to School or Child Care . . . when child feels better and temperature is normal for 24 hours.

Possible Diagnosis: **Scabies**

What You Should Know

- A parasitic infection caused by mites that burrow under superficial layer of skin
- Incubation period is up to 30 days
- Causes intense itching
- Often seen in moist areas of the body, such as groin, buttocks, webbed spaces of fingers and toes, and in underarms
- Burrows first appear as fine, gray lines under the skin; area of infection enlarges as adult mites burrow and lay eggs under the skin
- Diagnosed by skin scraping in which mite or egg is seen

- Transferred by close body contact and shared clothing
- Mites cannot jump or fly
- Child must be treated at home with prescription mite-killing cream or lotion
- Itching might last 2 to 4 weeks after treatment

What You Can Do As a Caregiver
- Notify child's parent
- Notify all other parents of a case of scabies, but maintain confidentiality
- Machine wash all washable items in hot water, including bed linens, blankets, towels, clothing, jackets, and hats
- Use hot setting on dryer
- Place pillows and stuffed animals in a dryer on hot setting for 30 minutes
- Leave items that cannot be washed or dried in a closed plastic bag for 4 days
- Vacuum upholstered furniture, rugs, and car seats
- Do not use mite sprays
- Discourage child from scratching

Child May Return to School or Child Care . . .
1 day after treatment is applied.

What You Can Do As a Parent
- Follow Caregiver recommendations
- Wear disposable gloves while treating with mite-killing lotion. Follow package directions.
- Wash hands thoroughly after removing gloves
- Bathe child 8 to 10 hours later to wash off lotion
- Check with child's health care provider about repeating full treatment in 1 week
- Do not use mite-killing lotion on infants
- Treat all infected family members at same time

Possible Diagnosis: Scarlet fever (Scarlatina)

What You Should Know
- A streptococcal bacterial infection that causes a generalized illness
- More serious than simple "strep" throat
- Incubation period is 2 to 5 days
- Contagious. Spreads from person to person by direct contact and by inhaling tiny droplets of infected secretions from nose.
- Signs and symptoms:
  - Rash appears primarily on trunk and is most intense at underarms, groin, behind knees, and on inner thighs
  - Rash resembles a sunburn covered with tiny "goosebumps"
  - Rash starts on chest and spreads downward
  - Painful sore throat
  - High fever
  - Tongue has white coating that changes to strawberry color after 4 to 5 days
  - Nausea and vomiting
- Skin peels after 1 week
- Treated with an antibiotic
- If untreated the child may be at risk for developing rheumatic fever

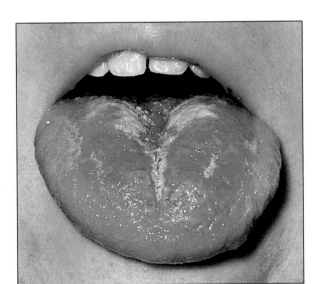

Scarlet fever

What You Can Do As a Caregiver
- Take temperature and treat for fever as necessary. Know your center's policy concerning the use of acetaminophen.
- Give throat lozenges
- Encourage clear fluids
- Wash hands thoroughly after caring for child to reduce chance of spreading infection to yourself and others
- Notify parent

Child May Return to School or Child Care . . .
24 hours after antibiotic treatment has started, when temperature is normal for 24 hours, and when child feels well.

What You Can Do As a Parent
- Wash hands thoroughly after caring for child
- Call child's health care provider

Sore Throat

Possible Diagnosis: Viral sore throat

What You Should Know
- Contagious
- Will get better without treatment
- More than 90% of sore throats are viral

What You Can Do As a Caregiver
- Take temperature and treat for fever as necessary. Know your center's policy concerning the use of acetaminophen.
- Wash hands thoroughly after caring for child
- Do not allow child to share mouthed toys, pacifiers, bottles, cups, or eating utensils

Child May Return to School or Child Care . . .
when temperature is normal.

What You Can Do As a Parent
- Follow Caregiver recommendations
- Call child's health care provider for throat culture if symptoms persist for more than 2 to 3 days

Possible Diagnosis: "Strep" throat

What You Should Know
- A streptococcal bacterial infection
- Occurs much less often than a viral throat infection but is more serious
- Abrupt onset
- Highly contagious. Spreads from person to person by direct contact and by inhaling tiny droplets of infected secretions from nose.
- Incubation period is 2 to 5 days
- Child is infectious only after symptoms appear and remains infectious until antibiotics have been taken for at least 24 hours
- Signs and symptoms:
  - Persistent, painful sore throat, especially when swallowing
  - White patches on throat and tonsils
  - Persistent fever
  - Swollen glands
  - Headache
  - Nausea and vomiting
- Can be serious, if untreated, possible later damage to heart and kidneys
- Requires throat culture to diagnose
- Treated with antibiotic
- Also see *Scarlet Fever* under *Skin Eruptions and Rashes*

What You Can Do As a Caregiver
- Take temperature and treat for fever as necessary. Know your center's policy concerning the use of acetaminophen.
- Wash hands thoroughly after caring for child
- Do not allow child to share mouthed toys, pacifiers, bottles, cups, or eating utensils

Child May Return to School or Child Care . . .
after 24 hours of antibiotic treatment and when temperature is normal.

What You Can Do As a Parent

- Follow Caregiver recommendations
- Complete course of antibiotic treatment to prevent relapse, even if child appears to recover quickly

Tooth Pain

Possible Diagnosis: Bottlemouth

What You Should Know

- Special form of tooth decay in very young children
- Caused by lengthy exposure to milk or other liquids containing sugar at naptime and bedtime
- Most common in upper front teeth
- Treatment often requires oral surgery with general anesthesia

What You Can Do As a Caregiver

- Do not give child a bottle of milk or juice (or any fluid containing sugar) at nap or bedtime. Give only water, or eliminate sleep time bottle.

Bottlemouth

What You Can Do As a Parent

- Follow Caregiver recommendations

Possible Diagnosis: Cavities

What You Should Know

- Caused by sticky foods that leave sugar coating on teeth
- Affects children age 3 and older

What You Can Do As a Caregiver

- Avoid sticky foods that cling to teeth and cause decay, such as raisins, gummy fruit-flavored treats, caramel candy, and licorice
- Encourage popcorn, pretzels, raw vegetables, fresh fruit, and yogurt
- Encourage child to brush teeth after snacks and meals. Use toothpaste with fluoride when child is old enough to spit it out instead of swallowing it.

What You Can Do As a Parent

- Follow Caregiver recommendations.

Possible Diagnosis: Teething

What You Should Know

- Gum pain caused by newly erupting teeth
- Can cause exaggerated crankiness
- Can be very painful and cause sleepless nights
- Can be accompanied by low-grade fever (< 102°F)

What You Can Do As a Caregiver

- Provide teething toys on which child can chew
- Do not rub child's gum with your finger
- Use over-the-counter topical teething products. Know your center's policy about the use of these products.
- Wear disposable gloves
- Wash hands thoroughly after removing gloves

Child May Return to School or Child Care . . .
child need not be excluded from child care or school.

Child May Return to School or Child Care . . .
child need not be excluded from child care or school.

Child May Return to School or Child Care . . .
child need not be excluded from child care or school if temperature is normal.

What You Can Do As a Parent
- Follow Caregiver recommendations
- Contact child's health care provider if fever exceeds 102°F because child might also have infection

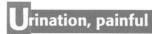

Urination, painful

Possible Diagnosis: Urinary tract infection

What You Should Know
- Infection usually caused by bacteria
- Signs and symptoms:
  - Strong burning sensation on urination
  - Feelings of frequent and urgent need to urinate
  - Urinating in small amounts
- More common in girls than boys because of short urethra and close proximity to anus

What You Can Do As a Caregiver
- Notify child's parent
- Encourage fluids
- Teach girls to wipe only from front to back after toileting

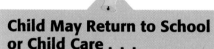

Child May Return to School or Child Care . . . child need not be excluded from child care or school.

What You Can Do As a Parent
- Follow Caregiver recommendations
- Call child's health care provider promptly
- Child needs to give urine specimen and be treated with antibiotic
- Avoid using bubble baths because these products can irritate urethra in boys and girls

Vomiting

Possible Diagnosis: Viral gastrointestinal infection

What You Should Know
- Many are contagious
- Less often caused by food poisoning or emotional upset
- Also see *Vomiting,* Chapter 16

What You Can Do As a Caregiver
- Wear disposable gloves when handling vomit
- Wash hands thoroughly after removing gloves
- Remove child from the group
- Notify parent
- Give no food or fluid until 1 hour after vomiting has stopped

Child May Return to School or Child Care . . . the following day if child feels better and temperature is normal.

What You Can Do As a Parent
- See *Vomiting,* Chapter 16

Additional Photo Credits

Chapter 1
Opener © Bob Daemmrich, Stock Boston
p. 5 © Ambu® Inc.

Chapter 2
Opener © Mark Gibson
p. 14 © Craig Jackson, In the Dark Photography

Chapter 3
Opener © Index Stock Photography and/or Jan Halaska 1998

Chapter 4
Opener © Mark Gibson

Chapter 5
Opener © Index Stock Photography and/or Charlie Borland 1998

Chapter 6
Opener © Melanie Carr, Zephyr Images

Chapter 7
Opener © Mark Gibson

Chapter 8
Opener © Index Stock Photography and/or Richard Wood 1998
p. 93 © Mark Gibson

Chapter 9
Opener © Zephyr Images

Chapter 10
Opener © Billy Barnes, Stock Boston
p. 113 © 1998 Jim Markham (top);

p. 113 © 1995 Wedgworth/Custom Medical Stock Photo (left);
p. 113 © S.J. Krasemann/Peter Arnold, Inc. (right);
p. 123 © 1998 Lance Beeny (left);
p. 123 © 1998 Grace Davies (right)

Chapter 11
Opener © Index Stock Photography and/or Dave Lissy 1998

Chapter 12
Opener © Index Stock Photography and/or Richard Wood 1998

Chapter 13
Opener © Zephyr Images

Chapter 15
Opener © James Darrell/Tony Stone Images

Chapter 16
Opener © Ken Fisher/Tony Stone Images

Chapter 17
Opener © Kevin Horan/Tony Stone Images

Chapter 18
Opener © Zephyr Images

Common Childhood Illnesses
p. 203 © Esbin/Anderson
p. 204 © Dr. H.C. Robinson/Science Photo Library
p. 206 © 1991 Keith/Custom Medical Stock Photo
p. 207 © Science Photo Library
p. 209 © William B. Chan, DMD, Tufts University, School of Dental Medicine

Index

Sports-related injuries, 93
Sprains, 90, 92
Stings
    insect, 46, 113, 115-117, 118
    scorpion, 121-122
Stitches. *See* Sutures
Strep throat, 166, 206-207
Sty, 198
Sunburn, 66, 68-69
Sutures, 54
Swallowed object, 82
Syrup of ipecac, 98, 99, 100

Teething, 207-208
Tetanus, 54
Thrush, 166, 201

Tick removal, 122-124
Tooth pain, 80, 207-208
Toy safety, 183

Urinary tract infection, 208

Viruses, 165-166, 198, 206, 208
Vomiting, 173-174, 208
Water safety, 186-187
Whooping cough, 194
Wounds, 51-57
    abrasions, 53
    infection of, 55
    lacerations, 53-54
    puncture, 54-55
    scalp, 53, 72